VAGUS NERVE STIMULATION:

MEDICAL TREATMENTS, SELF-HELP TECNIQUES AND EXERCISES FOR ANXIETY, DEPRESSION, TRAUMA AND AUTISM ACTIVATING THE NATURAL HEALING ABILITY OF YOUR BODY.

DAN SMITH

Table of Contents

Introduction

Breathing, digesting, regenerating, repairing, replicating, regulating—these are all processes undertaken by every organ in your body on a daily basis. When you think about it, it's truly amazing what happens in your body in just one day. In just 24 hours, your heart will beat 100,000 times. You will take 23,000 breaths. Your blood will circulate through your body three times every minute. During each of these cycles, your liver will cleanse and detoxify that blood. The culture of bacteria in your gut will break down food into the nutrients your cells need to live and grow (Habib, 2019). All of these processes are considered "automatic" brain functions, or functions that are directed without your brain having to consciously will them to happen. How amazing is that? With so much happening all the time, it would make sense that all of these processes are regulated by different parts of the brain and nervous system, all working together to ensure your body functions optimally, in peak health. And that's exactly how your body works to keep you healthy and whole. Right?

Wrong. All of the processes outlined above are managed, regulated, and activated by a single nerve, known as the vagus nerve. This single cord of bio-electrical signals begins in your brain stem (the highest point of the spinal cord) and branches out to almost all of your major organs. When it's not functioning properly, the effects can be felt in all areas of our health, from our mental wellness to the development of physical illness.

This book is a basic guide to understanding, healing, and activating the healing potential of this amazing nerve. The first part of this book will walk you through the science of the vagus nerve, with a basic introduction to your nervous system and its role as liaison between the organs of the body and the brain. Intimidating though this may sound, the language in this book will be broken down into simple, bite-size chunks that are easy to understand, whether you have a degree in neuroscience or barely made it through high school anatomy.

The middle section of this book will explain what can happen to us when the vagus nerve is not functioning properly. Sections will be devoted to the most common illnesses or disorders that we develop when the vagus nerve is not at optimum health. These sections will explain how and why the vagus nerve is connected to that (and similar) illnesses, as well as offer some basic solutions for how to prevent this kind of degeneration from happening within your own body.

Finally, the end of this book will be devoted to exercises you can do to activate the vagus nerve and stimulate its healing power. These exercises are for people of all ages and genders, as well as people at all different stages of health. No matter what illness, pains, or ailments you may have, these exercises are available to you to help you take back autonomy over your own wellness, and initiate the healing potential that you may not be finding in your medications or more conventional medical practices. If you feel you are in peak health and wellbeing, wonderful! These exercises aren't just for those who feel physically or mentally unwell. When incorporated into your daily routine, these exercises become simple acts of self-care that keep your vagus nerve (and therefore, the rest of your body) happy and healthy.

Chapter 1 What Is the Vagus Nerve?

Vagus is a derivative of the Latin word or "rambling, wandering or uncertain." The name was chosen due to the enigma of the vagus nerve. Anatomists can tell exactly what it is, but they know that the nerve wanders to many parts of the body.

The vagus nerve starts from the brainstem, the regulator of the autonomic nervous system. The brainstem senses, processes and regulates most of body's automatic functions. Automatic functions are the ones that our body performs automatically and unconsciously. Examples of automatic functions include:

- Sexual arousal
- Sweating
- Digestion
- Breathing
- Production of tears and saliva
- Detoxification of the kidney and liver
- Dilation of blood vessels
- Dilation of the pupils

The brainstems contain numerous groups of neurons called nuclei (nucleus for singular). The neurons are responsible for transmitting information to various parts of the body. They take information to and from the brain. There are two major types of neurons based on the direction information is being transmitted to. They are called afferent neurons and efferent neurons. Afferent neurons transmit information from the body to the brain while efferent neurons transmit information from the brain to other parts of the body. Efferent information, is information transmitted by efferent neurons are called consist motor and regulatory information.

Most of the nerves in the body carry simple motor signals or sensory information around the body. The vagus nerve performs much more than that. The left and right part of the vagus nerve contains four separate nuclei, each one with a different function. Of all the information carried by the neurons of the vagus nerve, about 20% are efferent information while the remaining 80% are afferent information. This means that most of the information in the vagus nerve is moving from the body to the brain. The vagus nerve transmits four times more information to the brain than it transmits away from it. Even with this, the efferent information it transmits is enough to have a huge impact on different organs.

Neurons are like a wired network, the information is transmitted like an electric signal which releases a chemical signal called neurotransmitter at the end of the line. The neurotransmitter then triggers an effect on the receiving cell by binding with a receptor on the receiving cell.

The vagus nerve mainly uses Acetylcholine (Ach), a neurotransmitter with an anti-inflammatory effect. This makes regulating inflammation a major function of the vagus nerve. In fact, the vagus nerve is the body's main manager of inflammation. Inflammation is the body's response to infections. It is a self-defense mechanism that sometimes gets out of hand. When inflammation becomes acute, it can lead to several health conditions. Some of the health conditions that may be caused by inflammation include:

- Diabetes
- High blood pressure
- Cancer
- Alzheimer's disease
- Heart disease
- Arthritis
- High cholesterol levels

All the organs affected in these conditions are connected to the Vagus nerve. It would be simplistic and dangerous to attribute these health conditions to the Vagus nerve and inflammation alone. There are many other factors that may contribute to these diseases but the contributions of inflammation cannot be ignored.

The Anatomy of The Vagus Nerve

The Brainstem- The Starting Point

The vagus nerve consists of neurons that begin at the brainstems. These neurons make up four nuclei. Each one of the nuclei control different fibers of the vagus nerve. The four nuclei are:

- Spinal trigeminal nucleus

Signals from the exterior part of the body transmitted through the skin by sensory neurons are transported through the vagus nerve by the spinal trigeminal nucleus.

- Nucleus solitarius (solitary nucleus)

Internal signals are transported by the vagus nerve to the nucleus solitarius (solitary nucleus). Internal signals are signals from internal organs such as the liver, intestine, heart, lungs, spleen, gallbladder, stomach and pancreas.

- Dorsal motor nucleus

The vagus nerve also sends signals to these organs through the dorsal motor nucleus. These signals control and regulate the aforementioned organs.

- Nucleus ambiguus.

The vagus nerve sends out neurons that possesses a motor function through the nucleus ambiguous. These neurons control most of the muscles in our upper airway and throat. They keep the airway open and vocal, ensuring our ability to speak/make sounds with our mouth.

The Neck

The fibers of the right and left sections of the vagus nerve extend from the medulla oblongata to the cranial cavity, where they converge into the vagus nerve. The vagus nerve exits the skull through the jugular foramen, a large opening between the skull and the neck that nerves and blood vessels pass through.

The vagus nerve leaves the skull for an area in the upper neck, behind the ear and between the internal carotid artery and internal jugular vein. Jugular/superior ganglion occurs as soon as the vagus nerve passes through the jugular foramen. It is the thickening of the vagus nerve by the sensory neuron cells. The cell bodies join to form a thinner nerve section, resulting in the first branch of the vagus nerve.

This branch is called the auricular branch. It returns to the skull through the mastoid canaliculus and comes back out of the skull and heads for the ear through the tympanomastoid fissure. It then extends through the skin of the ears. The auricular branch or the vagus nerve senses temperature, touch and moisture/wetness on the skin of the air, especially the auricle, tragus and external canal.

The vagus nerve thickens again to form the inferior/nodose ganglion, as it moves downward. The neurons in the inferior ganglion transmit information from internal organs.

The vagus nerve thins back and passes through a passageway made by the thickening of the carotid sheath (a connecting tissue).

The vagus nerve forms another branch in the in the carotid sheath. This new branch is called the pharyngeal branch. It contains neurons from the vagus nerve, the glossopharyngeal nerves (ninth cranial nerves) and the accessory nerves (eleventh cranial nerves).

The pharyngeal branch moves through the midline of the body until the reach the pharynx (the upper throat). Here, they release motor signals to the muscles responsible for opening and closing the mouth, gag reflex and swallowing.

The vagus nerve forms another branch called the superior laryngeal nerve as it moves down the carotid sheath on the sides of the neck. The superior laryngeal nerve transmits motor signals to the muscles that control the pitch of the voice and other muscles of the larynx, above the vocal chords.

The vagus nerve forms another branch called the thoracic cardiac branch. It is formed after passing through the carotid sheath in the chest. It supplies sensory signals to the heart. It mingles with some nerves of the nervous system to form cardiac plexus.

The Thorax

The vagus nerve continues downward into the thorax after leaving the carotid sheath. The left vagus nerve travels in front of the arch of the aorta and another laryngeal branch is formed. The right vagus nerve travels in front of the right subclavian artery and also forms a laryngeal nerve. Both laryngeal branches go upward, towards the neck. They transmit motor signals to the larynx muscles below the vocal cords. This helps to loosen and tension the vocal chords in order to produce sound.

Both the left and right vagus nerves send another branch to the lungs. The right vagus nerve sends a pulmonary branch to the posterior pulmonary plexus while the left vagus nerve sends a pulmonary branch to the anterior pulmonary plexus. They mingle with some neurons and connect to the bronchi on each lung.

The vagus nerve also transmits signals to and fro the thymus. The thymus is a vital part of the immune system that is located between the sternum and the heart. It is responsible for the training and growth of white blood cells. It develops early but may be covered by fat tissue as we age.

The Abdomen

The vagus nerve also innervates the abdomen, which aids digestion, detoxification and the entire immune system. The first branch extends to the stomach where it stimulates the stomach muscles for digestion. They also stimulate the stomach's muscle cells to push and churn the food and the parietal cells to produce hydrochloric acid (HCI), which is responsible for the secretion of digestive enzymes like gastrin and renin.

The second branch extends to the liver, where it may help generate hunger and craving for some nutrients. We absorb most macronutrients such as amino acid, carbohydrates, fat into the bloodstream in the small intestine. The nutrients then pass through the portal vein into the liver where they are filtered, detoxified and processed while the vagus nerve transmits signals to the brain. This signal involves details of fat intake, liver functionality, blood sugar level and quantity of bile needed in the digestion of fat.

The gallbladder holds the bile and bile salt created by liver in readiness of another meal. The vagus nerve helps the gallbladder pump the bile into the duodenum when we are eating. This process releases fat into the bloodstream. It is activated when the taste buds sense fat in the food.

Another branch is extended to the pancreas and transmits message to and fro the brain. The pancreas has endocrine and exocrine parts. The exocrine pancreas secretes digestive enzymes into the small intestine. The most popular of these enzymes are amylase (for breaking down carbohydrates), lipase (for breaking down fat), and protease (for breaking down protein). The endocrine pancreas balances the glucose levels by secreting glucagon and insulin into the bloodstream.

The vagus nerve transmits information about endocrine and exocrine cells from the pancreas to the brain. It also transmits information from the brain to the pancreas, about food content and the enzymes to be released into the digestive system and the bloodstream.

After the stomach, the parasympathetic fibers of the vagus combine with the lumbar sympathetic nerves to form the celiac plexus, a network that extends branches to the remaining organs of the abdomen.

It first branches into the spleen on the left side of the body, where it monitors the bloodstream and controls the immune system. The spleen shares the responsibility of controlling the immune system with the thymus until the thymus starts to disappear as we grow up.

Then it extends to the small intestine where it triggers the transportation of food down the tract. The digested food is passed into the small intestine where it undergoes further digestion. The vagus nerve triggers the smooth muscle cells of the gut to push a chyme (technical name for a bite of food) down the digestive tract.

The vagus also extends to the large intestine, where it transmits signals between the brain and the large intestine. The large intestine hosts the symbiotic bacterial that live in our gut. These bacterial produce biochemical precursors, minerals and vitamins. They also produce harmful gasses and toxins. The vagus nerve helps the body to keep the microbiome in check by transmitting information about the microbiome to the brain and instructions back to the large intestine.

Lastly, the vagus nerve extends into the kidneys. It helps the kidney to maintain pressure which is needed to filter fluid out of the body. The fluid is urine, a combination of water and uric acid.

The vagus nerve ends by combining with the parasympathetic nerves at the lower end of the spine. This network innervates the descending and sigmoid colon (the second half of the large intestine), the sex organs and the bladder.

Chapter 2 What Is the Polyvagal Theory?

In 1994, Dr. Stephen Porges, who was the director of the Brain-Body Center at Illinois University in Chicago, developed a unique perspective on the autonomic nervous system (ANS). Until that point, the ANS was thought to be comprised of two systems or response mechanisms: the sympathetic, action-initiating, and the parasympathetic, deactivating and calming nervous systems. Porges determined there is a third, extreme ANS response, which freezes and immobilizes the individual. He also determined that the vagus nerve, which is the 10th and longest, most diverse of the 12 cranial nerves emanating primarily from the brainstem, mediates or influences two of the three systems. One is the parasympathetic nervous system, which deactivates the action and energy of the sympathetic response, replacing it with a calming response system. This relaxing effect is mediated by a frontal branch of the vagus nerve, which Porges named the ventral vagal.

The rear branch of the vagus nerve, the dorsal vagal, is responsible for the primitive, shutting down and freezing responses to threats and extreme emotional and physical stress.

Porge's discoveries have the potential for both involuntary and voluntary actions that can affect our physical and mental states. Applications range from simple relaxation and calming techniques (that you can easily learn and put into daily practice) to professional medical treatment of diseases and disorders, among these are anxiety, depression, and Asperger's Spectrum, including autism. Polyvagal Theory applications include facial expressions and body language, as well as manual stimulation of the vagus nerve to achieve vagal tone. These can induce emotional responses, leading to the emergence of social engagement possibilities not previously attainable among autistic patients, especially children.

From an evolutionary standpoint, the sympathetic nervous system developed first as the body's urgent response to danger, frequently referred to as the fight or flight response. It is automatically and involuntarily activated when an imminent life and death, or otherwise serious threat, is perceived. Fifty thousand years ago, when our Homo Sapiens ancestors were confronted with a wild animal or an aggressive, potentially violent adversary, the sympathetic nervous system stimulated a rapidly elevated heart rate and breathing rate that increased blood pressure, while simultaneously suppressing the metabolism. These actions effectively shut down key visceral activities, including digestion, to divert energy to the more immediate situation. Hormones, including adrenaline, were released to increase energy stores for action further.

While our species today does not regularly confront life-threatening situations, our sympathetic responses remain ready to activate when stimulated by stress, frustration, anger, panic and anxiety. The same involuntary fight or flight mechanisms come into play and we can still get pumped up in any number of situations and confrontations.

More recently in our species' evolutionary history, the parasympathetic nervous system evolved as a counter to the sympathetic response, inducing relaxation by bringing down heart rate and breathing rate, lowering elevated blood pressure, reactivating the digestive system, and creating a sense of calm. Preparedness of fight or flight is replaced by what is called rest and digest. The body attains a state of homeostasis, or normality. The parasympathetic response is mediated by the ventral vagus nerve, which has branches reaching the heart, lungs, diaphragm and the entire digestive system.

Dr. Porges' work in developing the Polyvagal Theory led him to discover a third ANS response, called the freeze, mediated by another branch of the vagus nerve, called the dorsal, a nearly total shutting down of the individual's ability to react and respond. Interestingly, it may appear to be an overreaction of the sympathetic response's call to action, but Porges positions it as an extreme parasympathetic response of calming the body too much. The individual may enter a state of panic that prevents movement, speech, any action at all, freezing in place, immobilization, or fainting. Involuntary urination may occur, and the person might even go into shock, which, if severe and prolonged, may lead to cardiac arrest and death.

Among other mammals and reptiles facing a situation with no apparent escape, the response may be to freeze in place and play dead until the threat disappears, or an escape route becomes apparent. This playing dead act may be involuntary, being activated before the creature is even conscious of the situation.

Why Does It Matter to You?

One of the key breakthroughs of the Polyvagal Theory is the discovery that sympathetic responses may be brought under control voluntarily. Conditions ranging from anger, frustration, tension, and aggravation can be eased into a state of calm though mental and physical exercises. These exercises may be practiced alone, at home or while traveling, even at work if a quiet location can be found. Some find that stepping up the level of exercise is beneficial—cardiovascular training that can range from daily walks to more strenuous forms of working out.

If your concerns for your well-being extend beyond simply trying to stay calm and positive in the moment or if you are affected by extreme stress and anxiety, depression and more serious disorders, Polyvagal Theory applications may extend to professional massages and manipulation of the vagus nerves. Autistic patients may respond positively to facial expression and body language approaches that put them at ease, and enable social engagement not previously achieved through other methods and medications.

How Can It Be Applied?

The Polyvagal Theory has raised the level of credibility of a variety of physical and mental practices, bringing a scientific rationale to what was previously thought to be anecdotal, or suggestive results.

One particularly easy yet effective approach is managed breathing, the conscious control of inhales and exhales, the forceful extensions and contractions of the diaphragm, the addition of focused thoughts to drive out intruding negative thoughts. Other techniques include mindfulness, or being in the moment, a state of consciousness of the environment and its sounds, feelings and sensations.

Traditional practices, including Yoga and meditation, which have long been applied to achieve states of peace and calm, are now understood by Polyvagal Theory to apply physical stimuli to the ventral vagus nerve, initiating the parasympathetic response. Both Yoga and meditation emphasize managed breathing, and this practice alone is credited with initiating meaningful physiological and mental changes. Brain scans verify immediate and long-term changes in blood flow in the brain during meditation.

Yoga poses and stretches are also recognized to be encouraging what is called vagal tone, which are the signals to the organs to slow down, relax and achieve a lasting sense of calm. The same positive effects may be achieved by Pilates and other techniques that involve stretching and assuming poses that tense various muscle groups.

Persons whose condition is more serious can benefit from professional assistance. Chiropractic doctors working with Asperger's patients recognized that Polyvagal Theory is compatible with their salutogenic healthcare model, by supporting the recognition that the body can self-regulate itself and can self-heal under the right conditions. This inspired recognition that the Polyvagal can enable the doctors to tap into the healing potential. They apply neurological exercises that stimulate vagal tone in their patients. This empowers the Asperger's Spectrum patients with new ways to hear, to perceive, to respond to people and situations, to smile, to speak, to maintain eye contact.

On the medical level, electric stimulation of the vagus nerve is successfully being applied to treat epilepsy, notably in cases where the patient has not responded well to drugs. A small electrical device is implanted subcutaneously, and a thin wire extends to connect with the left vagus nerve. When spasm-inducing impulses are detected by the device, it emits an electrical pulse that stimulates the vagus nerve to send a signal to the brainstem, which in turn transmits the impulse to the part of the brain controlling involuntary seizures. To date, results are successful in up to 50% of cases.

Electrical stimulation is also being applied in cases of extreme depression that's not controlled by medication or electroshock therapy. Results in reducing depression have been mixed, and experimentation continues. Other conditions responding in some degree to electrical vagal stimulation include Parkinson's Disease, cluster headaches, rheumatoid arthritis, and irritable bowel disease.

Recently, non-invasive electrical vagus nerve stimulation devices (that do not require surgical implantation) have been developed, promising a wider range of possible applications. European authorities have authorized a range of applications. So far, in the U.S., testing has been mostly limited to treating cluster headaches.

Chapter 3 The Enteric Nervous System

The enteric nervous system is a system of nerves interconnecting the instinctive organs. We know alongside nothing about these nerves; since they are so joined with one another, with the instinctive organs, and with the connective tissue between the organs, it has been incomprehensible so far for anatomists to follow the pathways of the enteric nerves completely. Subsequently, we don't discover them very much spoke to in most life structures books. Moreover, we know nothing of how the enteric nerves work. Best case scenario, we can figure that the enteric nerves here and there help the distinctive instinctive organs to speak with one another to organize the complicated procedure of processing.

The Three Circuits of the Autonomic Nervous System

The autonomic nervous system comprises of three neural circuits:

- The ventral part of the vagus nerve (favorable conditions of unwinding and social commitment)

- The thoughtful spinal chain (battle or flight)

- The dorsal part of the vagus nerve (stoppage, shutdown, and burdensome conduct).

These three circuits direct our substantial capacities to help us look after homeostasis.

The Polyvagal Theory additionally displays another measurement to our under-remaining of the autonomic nervous system. The autonomic nervous system not just controls the capacity of our internal organs; these three circuits likewise identify with our excited states, which this way drives our conduct.

The Five Stages of the Autonomic Nervous System

Biobehavioral: the connection of conduct and organic procedures

In contrast to the old model of the autonomic nervous system, which concentrated solely on its guideline of the capacity of the instinctive organs, the new model relates every one of these three neural circuits with an enthusiastic state. Notwithstanding these three states, we have two cross breed expresses, every one of which joins two of the individual circuits, for an aggregate of five potential states of our autonomic nervous system.

The three neural pathways of the ANS:

The social-commitment nervous system. It includes movement in the ventral part of the vagus nerve (CN X) and four other cranial nerves (CN V, VII, IX, and XI). The ventral part of the vagus nerve identifies with positive feelings of delight, fulfillment, and love. As far as to conduct, it conveys what needs to be in positive social exercises with companions and friends and family.

The second of the ANS's neural pathways is the thoughtful spinal chain, which is initiated when our endurance is compromised. This condition of "preparation with dread" emerges when we are not protected or don't have a sense of security. The thoughtful spinal chain identifies with feelings of outrage or dread, which can convey what needs be in practices, for example, battling to defeat the risk or escaping to maintain a strategic distance from an undermining circumstance.

The third neural pathway is the dorsal part of the vagus nerve. This pathway is actuated when we face a mind-boggling power and fast approaching obliteration. When there is no reason for battling or fleeing, we con-serve what assets we have—we immobilize. Enactment of this pathway cultivates sentiments of helplessness, misery, and lack of care, showing in withdrawal and shutdown. This state can be portrayed as "immobilization with dread."

The fourth state is a half breed that supports the well-disposed challenge, or "assembly unafraid," which is suitable when we take part in focused games. This state consolidates the impacts of two neural circuits: the actuation of the thoughtful spinal chain enables us to activate ourselves to accomplish our best execution.

The fifth state is additionally a half breed of two neural circuits. Action in the dorsal part of the vagus nerve, when joined with that of the ventral part of the vagus nerve, underpins sentiments of closeness and private conduct. This state, which we could call "immobilization unafraid," is described by quiet, confiding in sentiments, permitting us, for instance, to lie still and nestle with a friend or family member.

A guideline is a term used to depict our capacity to deal with our passionate state, to quiet ourselves during times of uplifted feeling—when we become dreadful, profoundly dismal, irate, or baffled. The guideline is an educated procedure, one we coordinate into our own lives by watching others and, significantly, through the connection stages with our initial parental figures.

For instance, a newborn child may hear a noisy clamor or become scared by the uneven development of a pet that needs to play. The baby sees these little disturbances as potential dangers to his endurance. Incapable of "battle back" (or successfully stop the pet), the newborn child shouts out for a guardian to mediate and protect him from the circumstance. If the parent is receptive to the infant child, she will get the infant, give a physical grasp, and utilize mitigating language to help quiet the kid's neurological battle or-flight reaction.

These cooperation among parent and kid will shape the kid's capacity—or powerlessness—to control his feelings further down the road. This procedure is called co-guideline because of the parent steps in as a coach and outside wellspring of calming when the kid feels upset.

Chapter 4 Activating the Vagus Nerve

Divine Love, the universal energy from the Creator, exists everywhere in a neutral state. When you initiate a Petition, your Spirit activates the energy of Divine Love, and then your Spirit utilizes Divine Love to effect a change in your body. Your Spirit works with Divine Love unless you disconnect from Divine Love before your healing is complete. Should this occur, Divine Love returns to a neutral state, and nothing more happens until you reconnect your system to Divine Love. Now you understand the importance of always staying connected.

Harmful energy can exist in some or all of your energy layers. When dealing with a systemic blood disease or sepsis, it is likely that all layers have been contaminated by the harmful energy causing the illness.

For those of you exhibiting major inflammation in your body, you should note that there is a spiritual basis for this. Your spirit and mind interact and cause energetic and physical friction, resulting in inflammation (and sometimes swelling) that does not go away. People with weight control problems will see improvements when they use Petitions correctly to eliminate the inflammation in their bodies.

Occasionally, people report that their symptoms return after a few days. This usually occurs either because they stopped the petitions before healing was complete or they disconnected from Divine Love.

Staying Connected to Divine Love

- Let us first understand what is meant by accelerated healing. There are three fairly obvious factors to consider:

- When you have multiple illnesses, it should be obvious that it will take longer for you to heal than if you had just one straightforward problem. If you are very ill, it may take your body significant time to process the energy of Divine Love in your body.

- A person comfortable with our spiritual healing process and who has a single symptom frequently experiences instantaneous healing during a webinar. Others may take anywhere from hours to days to achieve the same level of healing, so please don't compare your progress to others. You are a unique individual, and your Spirit knows exactly what needs to be done.

- If you are distracted or become unloving towards yourself or others, you may unknowingly disconnect yourself from Divine Love, and then all healing ceases. Healing does not resume until you re-initiate that Divine Love connection.

By always staying connected to Divine Love, you will transition your entire system into a spiritual mode where you will be living a life of Divine Love. What does it mean to live life this way? Very simply, even when chaos erupts around you, you will be able to function without being driven by your emotions. And, you will be able to function with clarity while others become upset and lose their objectivity.

Also, each time you audibly state your intent to reconnect to Divine Love, you enable Divine Love to bypass any resistance to change that may come from your subconscious mind. This is vitally important to facilitate healing.

Remember that if you perceive that a physical symptom has left or is diminished, but it suddenly returns, it is quite likely that you have disconnected from Divine Love.

Feeling Divine Love Energy

If you are experiencing energy healing for the first time, you may not know the many ways Divine Love energy feels in your body. You might feel the heat, a tingle, a vibration, a cooling effect, or even see swirling energy around your body; it is all normal.

Since everyone has angelic support, some people find it more assuring to ask their Angels to assist them in processing Divine Love. Years ago, on our webinars, we always invited the Angels to participate. Now, with the energy of Divine Love so high,

Angelic participation is optional. Choose to work whichever way brings you the most comfort.

The simple act of accepting Divine Love fills your body with the right amount of Divine Love energy to heal your system. There is always enough Divine Love for the most complex healing, so you no longer need group support. You are self-healing in conjunction with the Creator's Divine Love.

Benefits

When you practice deep breathing techniques, you are going to benefit in many ways. Of course, the main why that you are going to benefit is by activating and stimulating your vagus nerve. This, of course, means that you are going to see all of the benefits of having a healthy vagus nerve, but there's even more.

1. Deep breathing is going to help to reduce stress and relieve anxiety.

2. It is going to help relieve pain. There are many techniques for deep breathing that focus completely on pain relief, and they work better as well as faster than any medication I have ever been given.

3. Deep breathing helps to improve a person's mood. It is actually a technique that is taught to children who have behavioral disorders as well as anger issues. Researchers understand that when we focus on our breathing and allow our bodies to stop that fight or

flight response, we are better able to control our own moods.

4. It helps to improve depression symptoms. One symptom that many people who have depression suffer from is a poor quality of sleep. However, when you practice deep breathing techniques, your quality of sleep is going to improve. It has also been found that deep breathing helps to reduce the heart rate of those that are struggling with depression as well as anxiety.

5. Deep breathing also helps to improve focus. Several studies have shown that by practicing deep breathing techniques for just 10 minutes, there was an immediate improvement of focus as well as a decrease in the person's blood pressure. Another study showed that by practicing deep breathing daily for just six weeks, test scores improved as well as rapid-fire test scores.

6. We spoke about OCD earlier in this book and how it is much more than just a desire to have a clean home. However, what we did not talk about is how hard OCD is to treat. The good news is that deep breathing techniques can help with OCD symptoms. In fact, studies have shown that practicing deep breathing patients' symptoms improve drastically even to the

point that they were able to reduce their medication dosages.

7. How many websites or eBooks have you seen lately that are focused on increasing one's energy? Maybe you have gone looking for a way to increase your energy. I have good news for you if you have any. Deep breathing exercises are going to help increase your energy levels. There is a very simple explanation for how this works. We already know that deep breathing helps to reduce stress, and it helps us to stay focused on the present. Because stress is reduced, the body has all of this energy that it was using by focusing on the stress, that is now freed up to be used for other things.

8. Deep breathing can actually help those that are suffering from obesity. Studies have shown that when a person uses deep breathing, they are able to overcome the hunger pangs that they struggle with when they are trying to lose weight or when they are fasting. We should have known this because how many times do, and we see monks fasting without looking as if they are starving to death? Sure, their bodies may be hungry, but they are taking control away from their body instead of letting it control them. By practicing deep breathing techniques, a person may find that they are better able to stick to

low-calorie diets or to fast without struggling with the hunger pangs that usually come with restricting food.

9. It helps with PTSD. There are so many people today that are suffering from PTSD for one reason or another. Some of our soldiers come home suffering from it, sometimes it is caused by a traumatic event that happened in childhood, but no matter what the reason deep breathing can help. When a person with PTSD practices deep breathing they are going to be able to sleep better, focus on what they are doing instead of getting distracted by the event that took place, they are going to be able to take control of the anger that they feel, and they will be less irritable.

10.   It can improve the quality of life of those that practice. There are so many benefits of practicing deep breathing that it is no wonder that research is showing that it can affect a person's entire life. What is even more amazing is that people often report feeling like they are finally experiencing life the way that it was meant to be experienced. They are able to focus on the tasks that they need to complete. Their productivity level increases dramatically. They are better able to get along with those around them. They begin focusing on their health, taking better care of themselves, and feeling better than ever before.

Is it really possible to change your life by doing something as simple as breathing? In short, yes. If you practice deep breathing techniques and you focus on doing them properly, you are going to see huge changes in your life. Remember, not only does deep breathing have its own benefits, but you are also going to see all of the benefits of stimulating your vagus nerve, which is what this is all about.

There are hundreds of different deep breathing techniques out there, many of them focusing on specific areas such as pain reduction or increasing energy. This means that you do not have to use the technique that I provided for you in this book. In fact, there are many guided, deep breathing techniques available for you to use online completely free. However, this was just an example for you so that you could see just how simple deep breathing is.

So come on, give it a shot. What do you have to lose? Deep breathing takes hardly any effort, and the benefits are so amazing.

Chapter 5 How To Know if Your Vagus Nerve Is Injured or Compressed

Your fringe nerves are the connections between your cerebrum and spinal rope and the remainder of your body. Fringe nerves are delicate and effectively harmed. Nerve damage can influence your cerebrum's capacity to speak with your muscles and organs. Harm to the fringe nerves is called fringe neuropathy.

Extending or pushing on a nerve can cause damage. The nerves additionally might be harmed because of other wellbeing conditions that influence the nerves, for example, diabetes or Guillain-Barre disorder.

In carpal passage disorder, weight on the middle nerve in the wrist causes harm. Or on the other hand the nerves might be squashed, cut, or harmed in a mishap, for example, games damage or an auto collision.

Now and then in a fringe nerve damage, either the strands or the protection are harmed. These wounds are bound to recuperate. In increasingly extreme fringe nerve wounds both the filaments and the protection are harmed, and the nerve might be totally cut. These kinds of wounds are exceptionally hard to treat and recuperation may not be conceivable. For instance, in the event that you feel shivering or deadness or create shortcoming in your leg, arm, shoulder or hand, you may have harmed at least one nerves in a mishap. You may likewise encounter comparative side effects if a nerve is being packed because of elements, for example, a limited path, tumor or different sicknesses.

It's critical to get restorative consideration for a fringe nerve damage as quickly as time permits since nerve tissue now and then can be fixed. Early analysis and treatment now and again can avert difficulties and lasting damage.

Signs Your Vagal Nerve Is Powerless

Vagal nerve sign can wind up feeble or the nerve can move toward becoming bothered because of overwhelming metal poisonous quality, poor stance, Hiatal hernias, abundance liquor, stress, and mind injury (a solitary blackout can cause powerless vagal nerve tone). Indications of powerless vagal nerve tone or misregulated terminating of the vagal nerve can cause the following manifestations:

- Lack of a muffle reflex

- Slow absorption: nourishment sits in your stomach excessively long. This can cause heartburn or GERD, swelling, or clogging.

- Inability to unwind

- Heart palpitations

- Insomnia

Probably the best indication of solid vagal tone is the point at which your pulse increases somewhat with inward breath, and moderate marginally with exhalation.

How Would You Reinforce the Vagal Nerve?

About 60% of vagal nerve tone is dictated by hereditary qualities; however, there is a strong 40% that we can affect! Become familiar with various approaches to fortify and animate the vagus nerve.

Fun truth: You CAN overstimulate the vagus nerve, and this is the most widely recognized reason for blacking out. On the off chance that you've at any point blacked out or felt tipsy in the wake of giving blood or getting a shot, you likely experienced "vasovagal syncope." At the point when you are under exceptionally high pressure your vagus nerve turns out to be excessively invigorated and your pulse drops rapidly making you feel woozy or lose cognizance. It's just brief, and sitting or resting for the most part settles the inclination rapidly.

Frail vagal nerve tone is connected to aggravation, wretchedness, forlornness and cardiovascular failures. We need to ensure our vagal nerves are solid! The following all invigorate the vagus nerve only enough to be exceptionally restorative, however less to cause blacking out but rather more these are not profoundly distressing occasions.

1. Gargling

Gargling animates the vagus nerve, albeit dainty swishing won't do it. You have to wash noisily and forcefully, to the point of nearly choking. Doing this day by day will help increment the responsiveness of your vagal nerve to direct unwinding, absorption, digestion, and that's just the beginning.

2. Playing Instruments

Fascinating research with didgeridoos demonstrated that playing the instrument is compelling in treating obstructive rest issue and rest apnea through its solid incitement of the vagus nerve. Further research demonstrates that various provocative conditions were additionally improved. Most wind instruments animate the vagus nerve.

3. Yogic or Deep Breathing

Holding your breath for 6-8 checks animates the vagus nerve. Attempt this: Use your stomach to take in for a check of 6, hold for 6-8, and breathe out gradually through pressed together lips for 6-8 tallies to get your vagus terminating. It's essential to have the option to feel your stomach (that line between your stomach and ribs) going all over with every breath. It takes around 10 minutes of this breathing to feel the profoundly loosening-up impacts of the vagal nerve incitement.

4. Meditation

Learning cherishing graciousness reflections improves vagal tone. This is because of its impact on positive feelings and positive associations. The more positive feelings and associations we have, the more grounded our vagal tone. Download my free reflection present.

5. Acupuncture

Acupuncture is astonishing for managing vagal nerve reaction. Electroacupuncture utilizes a little machine that emanates an effortless electromagnetic heartbeat. The electromagnetic heartbeat feels like a slight humming or tapping and isn't horrendous. Following 20-30 minutes of this, you will leave the workplace feeling unbelievably loose. That vagal nerve incitement will help direct every one of the procedures constrained by the vagal nerve, which at this point you know is a whoop dee doo!

Bioelectronics is a developing field of medication where little gadgets are embedded to animate diverse sensory system pathways. This effectively treats a scope of maladies and provocative side effects. This is energizing and approving of needle therapy which uses needles and other things to invigorate the sensory system at various focuses to treat a scope of illness and incendiary side effects. On the off chance that you need to be on the bleeding edge of logical research, and stay away from medical procedure to embed a metal gadget, attempt the less intrusive way, needle therapy.

Chapter 6 Vagus Nerve Stimulation

The theory of vagus nerve stimulation was in 1988 by a physician in the United States, Jacob.

According to Zabarra, he believes that stimulating the vagus nerve may change the potential in the brain, thus blocking or even preventing the onset of epilepsy.

As for why the stimulation of the vagus nerve can produce the effect of controlling seizures, there is no real conclusion yet, but it has been found in animal experiments.

Stimulating the vagus nerve is indeed effective in controlling the onset of epilepsy. This idea was later designed by Cyberonics to be a neurostimulation system called Neurocybernetic.

Prosthesis System (NCP), and is actually used clinically in patients with epilepsy.

The actual progression of vagus nerve stimulation is such that the coil is first placed surgically on the vagus nerve in the left neck and the stimulation device is buried in the chest, and then at each patient visit, the medical staff.

The instrument adjusts the parameters and modes in the stimulation device, and the machine automatically stimulates the vagus nerve according to the set mode to achieve the purpose of controlling seizures.

If the patient's seizure is a precursor, when the patient feels a precursor in the home or other places, you can use a small structure containing a magnet inside, and pass it across the chest to generate additional stimulation.

To interrupt an upcoming seizure, or to reduce the time of onset, or to reduce the severity of the episode

How To Stimulate the Vagus Nerve

So far, researchers have used a device that releases current to stimulate the vagus nerve, but there are other ways to do this. The vagus nerve genes of different tensions have a genetic predisposition, and through continuous practice, the tension level can be changed by the following method.

1. Humming

The vagus nerve is connected to the vocal cords, and the system's singing and humming sounds stimulate the nerves. You can try to sit quietly and repeat the sound of "OM".

2. Speaking

Similarly, the more people who speak, the more likely they are to increase their vagal tone through the sound, In general, singing and laughing will also work.

3. Wash your face with cold water

Cold water seems to stimulate the vagus nerve. When your body needs to adapt to the cold, the sympathetic nervous system will decline and the "reaction and digestion" system (parasympathetic nervous system) will increase. In other words, any sudden cold exposure increases the activation of the vagus nerve. You can do this by washing your face with cold water or taking a cold shower.

4. Take a deep breath with the diaphragm

Deep breathing from the diaphragm can stimulate and regulate the vagus nerve.

5. Yoga

Studies have shown that yoga and breathing exercises can significantly increase your vagal tone.

6. Meditation

According to a 2010 study, people who often meditate and think positively tend to have better vagus nerves.

7. Increase good intestinal bacteria

While the benefits of increasing gut-healthy bacteria are numerous, it is surprising that this also helps to establish a positive "feedback loop" through the vagus nerve, thereby increasing its tension. Probiotics are a source of healthy bacteria.

How To Stimulate the Vagus Nerve Naturally

How to stimulate the vagus nerve naturally - How to activate the vagus nerve to regenerate the body

ACTIVATE VAGUS NERVE WITH FOOD

The link between the vagus nerve and food goes beyond its innervation in the digestive system.

The intestinal flora or microbiota, is a set of millions of bacteria that are responsible for helping to digest food and assist in a huge variety of functions, among which is influencing our preferences about food and visceral emotions that they drive some of our actions.

This thanks to its role in the alkalinization or acidification of the intestinal environment that is perceived through the vagus nerve and interpreted as healthy and harmonic or unwanted, and can also damage the vagus nerve itself.

A correct diet allows the vagus nerve to function better and also, our emotional and digestive health is harmonized.

It is important to avoid or reduce:

- Flours and simple carbohydrates

- Pastries and refined sweets

- Sucralose or Splenda

- Dairy animals

- Processed meats

On the other hand, the intake of the following foods should be maintained or increased:

- Green vegetables

- Papaya

- Figs

- Garlic and Onion

Other Ways To Stimulate the Vagus Nerve

Enjoying a healthy relationship is another key to maintaining vagal health. In fact, people with better vagus tone are known to be more altruistic, closer and more harmonious.

This is because vagus nerve stimulation causes the release of oxytocin, a hormone called a "connecting molecule", to promote binding. Oxytocin is associated with human characteristics such as loyalty, empathy, trust and courage.

In this sense, research has found that there is a cycle of positive feedback between physical health that began to move through awareness of social connections, positive emotions, and vagal tension.

JOKE WITH FRIENDS

Therefore, one way to stimulate the vagus nerve is to meet a laughing friend. While laughter strengthens the relationship, it increases heart rate variability. This is a reliable indicator of the health function of the vagus nerve.

Finally, it is worth mentioning another way to stimulate the vagus nerve: via supplements.

Some supplements such as ginger root, probiotics (especially Lactobacillus rhamnosus), essential omega-3 fatty acids (especially DHA), and zinc can improve the health and function of the vagus nerve.

- Hold your breath.

- Place a fresh, damp cloth on your face.

- Press your eyes strongly.

- Drink a glass of cold water

- Lie down with your head down.

- Abdominal contraction

- Inflate the abdomen and send oxygen to the blood, deeply stimulating.

- Relaxation and meditation

The result of this stimulation can be surprising when you feel it or practice it at the moment of stress.

In addition, long-term stimulation of the vagus nerve reduces the repair of some organs, lowers blood pressure, improves heart rate, increases brain volume, improves immune function, repairs the nervous system, anxiety, stress, and depression.

Chapter 7 Turning Your Vagus On

What do nervousness, fractiousness, acid reflux, and restlessness share?

And when you said pressure, you're in good shape. More explicitly, they all derive from an absence of Vagus action. This sort of Vagus is significant to your wellbeing and prosperity.

You need to realize why your Vagus nerve is so basic and how to actuate it to quiet your nerves, rest and condensation better, and bolster your body's characteristic healing powers.

Your Vagus nerve interfaces your cerebrum with your heart, gut, and all your inner organs. Truth be told, its impact is unavoidable to the point that it has been designated "the skipper" of your parasympathetic sensory system, which is your body's characteristic unwind, remake, and fix reaction group.

Appropriate working of your Vagus nerve holds incessant irritation under tight restraints, putting the brakes on every significant sickness. It directs your heartbeat, amplifying pulse inconstancy, which is a significant marker for heart wellbeing.

Furthermore, it flags your lungs to inhale deeply, taking in the oxygen that renews your essential vitality.

Your Vagus nerve additionally deciphers fundamental data from your gut to your cerebrum, giving you gut impulses about what is useful or destructive for you. At that point, it encourages you to combine memories, so you recall significant data just as your well-meaning goals.

Finally, your Vagus nerve discharges acetylcholine, which counters the adrenaline and cortisol of your pressure reaction, and enacts your body's common Relaxation Response, with the goal that you can relax, rest, and let go.

Thus, presently, you have an image of why actuating your Vagus nerve is so basic.

The issue is that our present culture urges us to be so hyper-occupied, so hyper-invigorated, that we keep running in pressure mode, basically constantly, without knowing it. We are so used to incitement that we don't have the foggiest idea what genuine relaxation feels like, considerably less how to do it.

Rather than rehearsing a characteristic beat among action and rest, we are hyper-dynamic. What's more, we are so molded that we feel regretful if we're not continually accomplishing something, or exhausted if we're not being animated and engaged!

Accordingly, nervousness, peevishness, and restlessness are steady mates. This keeps us from resting profoundly and sets us on the way for ceaseless ailments, for example, malignant growth.

Things being what they are, how might we break this behavior?

Luckily, your body is profoundly strong. It is simply hanging tight for you to enact your normal parity, and that is as close as a couple of moderate, full breaths away.

At the point when you inhale gradually and deeply, your Vagus nerve is enacted. It sends quieting signals that moderate your brainwaves and pulse and set moving all the rest and fix systems of your body's regular Relaxation Response.

Along these lines, slow profound breathing is imperatively significant. Be that as it may, there's an issue. Living in steady pressure mode advances an example of limited, fast, shallow relaxing.

In this way, slow profound breathing may take a little practice. Here's an incredible method to do that.

A Simple Deep Breathing Meditation:

Lie on your back and gently close your eyes. Rest your hands, one over the other, on your lower stomach area.

As you breathe in, enable your lower guts to delicately rise, as though it is topping off with your breath. As you breathe out, enable your lower mid- region to unwind downwards, as though it is purging out.

Sink into a decent, simple cadence, daintily following your breath, as your stomach tenderly rises and falls. Check whether it's conceivable not to constrain it, just simply focus as it happens normally, effectively, easily.

As you proceed, check whether you can see the minute you start to breathe in and time it right until you normally stop. At that point, see the minute you start to breathe out and time it right until you normally stop.

Appreciate this calming beat, and after a couple of minutes-and afterward, see how great you feel.

And when you can, feel free to try this out, so you experience it for yourself...

You can rehearse this straightforward profound breathing reflection once per day to discharge the pressure of the day, and the layers of strain gathered from an earlier time. You can do it lying in bed around evening time before sleep to set up your body to rest deeply.

In a matter of moments, you'll have reset your body's regular parity, and this will convert into living an increasingly adjusted, happy, and tranquil life.

Chapter 8 Functions of the Vagus Nerve

The vagus nerve is responsible for the major organs in the body. But, let's talk about some of the more unique functions of the vagus nerve, what they are, and why they matter so much.

Natural Inflammation Treatment

Inflammation can be treated with the vagus nerve. It can also prevent inflammation as well. When you get injured, whether it be a cut, scrape, or anything else, you will notice some redness on the surface of your skin. This is totally normal.

But, if you notice that you have too much inflammation, this can be the cause of certain diseases and conditions. Some of these conditions or diseases include autoimmune disorders, celiac disease, rheumatoid arthritis, even sepsis can be the causes for too much inflammation, and your vagus nerve is part of the cause. The vagus nerve has a network of fibers that are all near your organs. Whenever there is an inflammation present, immediately the brain will get anti-inflammatory neurotransmitters to help control the immune response. But, if your vagus nerve isn't working properly, or if it's overstimulated, it can affect the severity of the inflammation which may cause certain conditions to exist for far longer.

Gut-Brain Communication

The vagus nerve is also where the brain and the gut communicate with one another. For example, if you ate something that didn't taste good, your vagus nerve will send a signal to the brain telling it that you don't want to eat whatever it was. Sometimes, if you're anxious about something, that funny feeling you get in your stomach is attributed to the nerve. Your vagus nerve is responsible for all that communication.

But, it does so much more than that. The vagus nerve also communicates your immune response. For example, if you eat something that you're allergic too, you'll experience inflammation, and as mentioned earlier, the vagus nerve, in communication with the brain, will step in to get the neurotransmitters to come forth, and from there clean everything out. Your vagus nerve will put everything in its rightful place. However, sometimes this may lead you to developing other allergies.

Controls Our Breathing

Breathing is a big part of our lives. The purpose of breathing isn't just simply to take in air; it's also important because it helps bring oxygen to our organs. Without oxygen, and without supplying our vital organs with it, we risk not being alive. However, sometimes breathing into much air can end up hurting us later on. You've probably been in a situation where you take in short but quick breaths of air; this often happens when you're anxious or nervous.

The vagus nerve also helps with relaxation. After a long day, I'm sure the first thing you want to do is sit on your couch and relax. The vagus nerve sends a signal to your body telling it that it wants to relax. As a result, the vagus nerve will also communicate to your diaphragm; the diaphragm will expand, thereby allowing more air into your system. This will help you feel more relaxed as you're able to take in longer and deeper breaths.

Have you ever noticed after taking deep breaths, especially while meditating, you feel more relaxed? That's because the vagus nerve is at play. It communicates with the body to help you feel more relaxed. It can help with anything from an anxiety attack to even just getting into a deep sleep after a long day. Those who practice meditation will notice that their bodies become incredibly relaxed due to deep breathing exercises.

The vagus nerve also plays a role in lowering your blood pressure and heart rate. The vagus can control your heart rate and how much blood gets pumped throughout your body. It will help regulate the necessary areas in your body so that your heart and blood pressure remain at an optimal level. Levelling out your heart rate and blood pressure will also help with cardiovascular health.

But, when the vagus nerve is overactive, it will cause the heart to pump too much blood. As a result, your heart will be working harder than it is used to. A rapid heart can lead to damage of other organs as well as loss of consciousness. Along with this, your blood pressure will also shoot through the roof, potentially leading to organ failures.

Vagus Nerve and Fear

Fear is something we all experience at some point. If we've ever been in a situation where we've felt fearful, the vagus nerve is at play in those cases. When you feel scared, your vagus nerve will send that information straight to the brain. Your brain will then accept the signal sent from the vagus nerve and warn you. As a result, your fight or flight response is triggered.

Going back to your gut, when you feel a pitfall in your stomach or an uncomfortable sensation, the vagus nerve is likely at play. If you continue to be fearful in a situation, your vagus nerve will register this information and bring back feelings of fear in other similar situations. An overstimulated vagus nerve can lead to anxiety and other problems in the body. A properly working and stimulated vagus nerve will determine how you respond to situations in life.

Vagus Nerve and Memory

Did you know the vagus nerve can also help with memory? A study conducted at the University of Virginia showed that when you stimulate the vagus nerve, memory was in turn strengthened (Adelson, 2004). This is because when the vagus nerve is properly stimulated, it sends signals to the brain of a lot of different things that are happening.

When you recall something, you release the neurotransmitter called norepinephrine deep into the amygdala, which is where our memories are stored. This could also account for why you experience an uncomfortable gut feeling when you're afraid, because the vagus nerve records the information of how you feel when scared and can recognize when you are scared again.

Our Natural Pacemaker

If you've never heard of a pacemaker before, or have never seen one, it's essentially a small device placed near your heart which sends out electrical signals directly to the heart to help it push out impulses. However, we already have a natural pacemaker in our bodies; therefore, not necessarily needing additional devices. The natural pacemaker is in the right atrium, located on the right side of the heart, which is where the acetylcholine is released and controls your pulse. You can measure your heart rate by keeping track of the number of beats. This will show your heart rate variability. The vagus nerve takes this information and then determines whether or not it needs to encourage the heart to pump more blood. So, the vagus nerve doesn't just help your heart rate but it also provides the heart with all the necessary information it needs to work its magic.

Controls Relaxation

The relaxation response is all thanks to the vagus nerve. If you feel the sensations of the fight or flight response from the sympathetic nervous system, then your vagus nerve will alert your body to relax. Your vagus nerve is responsible for pumping out acetylcholine, which is the hormone that tells your body to relax. The sympathetic nervous system pumps out cortisol and adrenaline, while the vagus nerve does the opposite.

What's amazing about this is that it can tell so many parts of your body to relax when it's experiencing high levels of stress. Imagine the vagus nerve as a control center, whereby it is in control of all the different parts of the body. It sends out signals to different areas of the body whenever enzymes or proteins need to be released. Some of the different chemicals your vagus nerve secretes include vasopressin, which helps with water loss; oxytocin, which helps with pain relief; and prolactin, which helps with milk secretion and promotes sexual potency. The vagus nerve controls a lot of the hormones within the body, hence why it's so important for us.

Monitors Our Gag Reflex

Your gag reflex is also stimulated by the vagus nerve. If something is going down the wrong pipe, your vagus nerve will immediately stimulate your gag reflex, causing you likely to cough. This cough reflex can also be stimulated through our ear canal. When there's something that shouldn't be in the ear canal, chances are your cough reflex will react and you will be forced to cough. These reflexes also ensure that your body is safe and secure, free of anything harmful.

Sweat Control

The vagus nerve also controls sweat, or lack thereof. When the body gets too hot, your vagus nerve will tell the body to secrete sweat to help cool it down. You may also experience excessive sweating whenever you're scared. Sometimes, sweating is a sign that you probably should leave the situation you're currently in. The vagus nerve, while also controlling your heart rate and your hormones, is also important for stimulation of the sweat glands in your body.

Stimulates Peristalsis

Finally, the vagus nerve can help stimulate peristalsis. Peristalsis is the contraction as well as relaxation of muscles that help push things forward. For example, when you swallow food, the muscles in your esophagus are constricting and relaxing to help push the food down to your intestines and stomach; this is what peristalsis is. In essence, it's a slow, pulsating motion which pushes contents. This is also where the vagus nerve can stimulate the gallbladder to form bile. Bile is produced from the broken down food. Peristalsis is something that happens in the digestive tract. If peristalsis does not function the way it's supposed to, or if you experience trouble with your bowels, this might be the cause of the food you ate and how it was digested. There are a few different types of disorders that this can cause if the vagus nerve isn't properly stimulated, but we'll get into those later.

The vagus nerve is responsible for a lot of different things that can happen in the body; therefore, when you're looking to improve the health of the vagus nerve, these various functions should all be considered, and understanding their functions is just as important.

Chapter 9 The Healing Power of Vagal Tone

The Polyvagal Theory has effectively linked the physical and emotional. Physical actions can regulate emotional conditions, emotional activities can cause physical responses. For example, deep, forceful, diaphragmatic breathing can initiate a state of deep calm, while emotional reactions can lead to stress, triggering elevated heart rate and respiratory rates and a range of other visceral organ reactions, such as stopping digestion to conserve energy. Given the role of the vagus nerve in mediating both physical and emotional reactions, it is no surprise that the vagus nerve can be engaged to better manage our emotional sense of well-being and help alleviate physical problems.

As we have seen, under normal conditions, the calming parasympathetic nervous system is dominant, keeping the body in a state of homeostasis. In this context, vagal tone is an assessment of the body's readiness to perform certain key functions effectively. An ideal vagal tone maintains a baseline from inputs, via the vagus nerve, received from the parasympathetic nervous system. Among the most important vagal tone functions is controlling heart rate to keep it from beating too quickly. Vagal activity is key as well to controlling breathing rate, managing the rate of peristaltic contractions during digestion, and further affecting the sensitivities and inflammation of the digestive tract and functioning of the liver.

Vagal tone is also a measurement of emotional stability, as emotions are at their baseline of normalcy when the dorsal vagal and ventral vagal responses are at homeostasis.

But this is not always the case, especially when emotional reaction ignite physiological responses.

Regulating Emotion

The parasympathetic nervous system follows two pathways. The better known, and far more dominant, is the ventral vagal pathway that controls most of the key organ functions. As noted above, it encourages social engagement and interaction to further secure and stabilize the individual. The more recently recognized but older pathway, the dorsal vagal, controls the emergency freeze response, which causes immobility, lightheadedness, speechlessness, fainting and shock. While the ventral vagal parasympathetic response is mediated by the neocortex, the newest and most developed part of the brain, the dorsal vagal parasympathetic response is mediated or activated by the most primitive, reptilian part of the brain.

Malfunctioning of either of these vagal pathways can lead to emotional disturbances, but regulating the vagal tone can moderate the disturbances. Brain function, specifically emotional responses and reactions, are directly affected by signals carried by the vagus nerve. Studies have shown that behavioral measures of emotional expression, emotional disturbances, self-regulatory skills, and reactivity may be correlated with baseline cardiovascular levels of vagal tone, leading to the conclusion that cardiovascular vagal tone can be an indicator of how well emotions are being regulated and managed. This perspective was not under consideration traditionally until the Polyvagal Theory opened this enlightened perspective and continues to encourage further experimentation.

The higher the level of vagal tone, the healthier the baseline condition of mind and body. Therefore, given the direct relationship between physical and emotional conditions, it follows that practicing the exercises to improve physical vagal tone will contribute to the improvement of emotional conditions, returning them to more normal baseline levels.

Emotional conditions that may be the consequence of low vagal tone include anxiety, depression, sensations of stress, fatigue not caused by excessive activity, and sleeplessness. Other, more long lasting emotional conditions may include Post Traumatic Stress Disorder (PTSD), and Attention Deficit Hyperactivity Disorder (ADHD). While many of these emotional disorders may respond to professional counseling and prescribed medication, hard-to-treat cases may respond favorably to vagal toning activities.

Practicing mindfulness, or being in the moment, is a variation on meditation, with awareness of every environment stimulus.

The effectiveness of all of these exercises can be enhanced by managed, diaphragmatic breathing, with deep, deliberate, thoughtful inhales and exhales, which directly stimulate the vagus nerve. The effect is to slightly increase the heart rate on inhales, and them to lower heart rate back to a healthy, or homeostatic baseline on exhales.

When vagal tone is high, physical and emotional states are normal. Low vagal tone, the consequence of not stimulating the vagus nerve, can result in the range of emotional disorders we've been discussing and, additionally, can contribute to a sense of apathy, loneliness, isolation, and negative moods. These are all symptoms of the inability to engage socially and participate in social interaction. This may continue a self-perpetuating downward spiral, with the sense of isolation tending to discourage social interaction, and with the disconnection from social engagements furthering the feelings of isolation.

Low vagal tone can have equally serious consequences physically, including cardiovascular disorders.

Cardiovascular Applications

The relationship between the vagus nerve and the heart has been extensively researched and verified, with further clarification emerging from the Polyvagal Theory.

To set the stage for understanding this relationship, let's begin with the physical side of the relationship, keeping in mind that the vagus nerve is neither organ or muscle, but is a long, multi-branched network of wire-like nerves connecting the brain and other organs, carrying the electrical impulse messages between them. This is how the vagus nerve carries messages that affect one of the most important physical elements, the heart, and does so every second, 24 hours every day.

The vagus nerve travels from the brainstem and connects with the heart muscle or myocardium on the upper right side of the heart, in a cluster of nerves called the sinus node, for short, or sinoatrial node. Here the vagus nerve acts like a natural pacemaker, regulating the heartbeat. During normal conditions, at times of homeostasis, when there is little or no activity or stress, signals arriving from the brain through the vagus nerve slow the heart rate to less than 100 beats per minute. It is subsequently slowed and regulated, sequentially, by the atrioventricular node, the bundle of His, the right and left bundle branches, and finally the Purkinje fibers at the bottom of the myocardium. Every second or so, the heart muscle contracts, blood is forced out of the ventricles toward the lungs from the right ventricle, and into the aorta from the left ventricle.

Now, here is where the relationship between the heart and emotional reactions occur, but first, a quick background. The Polyvagal Theory has added clarity to our understanding of how the autonomic nervous system in primates evolved from the more primitive reptile nervous system. Changes evolved to accommodate the more complex primate nervous system, resulting in increasingly elaborate vagal pathways that control or regulate the heart. There was a transition from the exclusive dorsal vagus nucleus among reptiles to a more elaborate structure in mammals, called the nuclear ambiguus.

This included a connection between the heart and the face that enabled social interactions to influence the visceral or bodily functions, and possible dysfunctions. In simple terms, this means that social activity and other emotionally-regulated activities could play a role in maintaining control over the heart rate, while conversely, cardiovascular events can directly affect the emotions.

Charles Darwin, the founder of evolutionary theory, recognized the bi-directional flow between the brain and the heart that is mediated by the vagus nerve. Darwin understood that facial expressions were a physical manifestation of emotions, and correctly surmised that there were neural pathways connecting the brain with the heart and other organs that would facilitate physiological responses to emotions. Darwin and those of his time were correct in their estimate, despite not yet knowing that the pneumogastric nerve, later renamed the vagus nerve, had its own private network connection between the brain and the heart, apart from the connections of the action-oriented sympathetic nervous system. Capabilities to elevate and reduce heart rate coexist.

Today, Polyvagal Theory has led to discoveries of how vagal tone, the state of homeostasis, can be determined. A simple but effective determination of vagal tone is measurement of the heart rate during inhalation, when it should increase slightly above baseline, and then, measurement of the heart rate during exhalation, when the heart rate should return to baseline. The different rates of the two heart rates can be used to specify the precise vagal tone.

What does this mean to you?

During times of stress, your physical side may be in a state of elevated heart and respiratory rate, and you may be sweating, feeling a need to exert yourself and take action. In those situations when the cause of the sympathetic response is alleviated, and there is no need to run, or fight, or jump, you can bring things down, calm your body, with thoughts of calm, peace, reassurance. Repeat to yourself that everything is cool, under control, and it's okay to relax.

On a more serious medical level, when controlling heart rate and respiration are beyond the self-application of physical and emotional exercises, a relatively new treatment is the subcutaneous insertion of a vagus nerve stimulator. It is connected to the vagus nerve, and generates regular electrical impulses, acting like a pacemaker to increase vagal tone. Newer technologies have led to non-invasive electrical stimulators that make access to this treatment less expensive, and enables application to a wide range of symptoms. One of the first successful applications of electrical vagus nerve stimulation has been treatment of epilepsy, and up to 50% success in reduction in seizures has been achieved, among patients not responding to medication.

Chapter 10 Integrating the Nervous System

At all stages, the nervous system must be soothed, incorporated, and trained. The autist will start engaging and directing the organ. The more that an autist can acquire knowledge of what is occurring, the more power they can achieve; so influence comes with understanding. By fact, we want autists to return to their bodies: to learn to direct them, rather than ad hoc running the system. We want to teach them to connect with their bodies and have more power. They can begin to learn to steer their body on a very simple, practical level as they begin to learn control. What we want to do is to get the nervous system out of the learnt pattern; to actually shore up the relationship between the social engagement process and the nervous system; and to build a bigger range of social cues. They want to reinforce the willingness of the autist to urge the body to settle down and tell the mind to re-engage and try something different at every moment. We can teach autists to be friends with their bodies, to understand and re-educate their learned patterns.

Living is an articulated experience, and a personal journey of exploration and mastering is reframing autism. To listen to the body, the autist must learn. Usually, this is a job done as babies. It's sluggish and the emphasis is on learning, communicating and re-integrating. It's fragile. It's not accomplishment-oriented, though the milestones can be fantastic when learned. Autism may not be a disease in neurobiology. It can be a learned response to trauma or an irritated vagal system by the autonomic nervous system. If so, the road ahead is to re-educate the body, re-inform the body, not just the mind, which takes more to heal than just a' snap out of it.' You can't just teach social skills to autists, or how to tie their shoelaces, because you/they must also teach their nervous system. They've got to train it to settle down and they've got to train it to include something, to wake up. It's not just about science, because the body and the brain need to be retrained.

Eventually, there has to be a stronger connection between body and brain, and that is immediately feasible with what we now learn regarding brain plasticity. The gift of neuroplasticity (the ability of the brain to rewire and create new circuits at any age as a result of input from our environment and conscious intentions) is that we can create a new level of mind. Dr. Joe Dispenza, DC They people have become very wise lately. We figured out we could adjust our minds and make them work a lot better. We've began to step into a whole new paradigm of seeing who we are as human beings and what we can do. Plasticity in the neuro (brain) is an exciting new research field. We find that the brain is open to all kinds of influences and can be re-wired. We already know that the brain will create new neurons and develop new neural pathways of all sorts. It is now necessary to relax, wake up and restore what was not functioning in the brain. The minds are garden-like.

We can plant new things, water them, and make them come alive. We used to believe that our minds, like a clock, were programmed and we just got what we were born with. We already know it's not true. Now we know our brains are organic; they grow and change continuously. Through new experiences, our minds shift, and if we want, we will make all sorts of different neural connections whether we are eight or eighty. We are starting to learn how easy it is to make changes. Stroke patients, people with chronic learning disabilities, feel that different cognitive interventions can enable significant changes in their lives. Since the fifteenth century, research has understood that the brain would alter, but it wasn't until recently that we as a group actually started to believe in its ability. Individual scientists have been investigating brain plasticity for hundreds of years, but they have never been taken very seriously by anyone in the science community, so consequently we have not.

It wasn't until the 1960s that trends started improving. Paul Bach-yRita devised an experiment in 1969 with a large camera, an electrically induced chair and plenty of wires and instructed congenitally blind people to recognize an image of the Twiggy supermodel. He wanted them to' think' ultimately. He had worked out how to teach new signals to the brain, to teach them how to convert tactile (feeling) information into visual information. It worked, and we realized just how much the brain works on physical and electrochemical images and signals. This research helped us understand that we are not built like robots, that our minds are simply packets of electrical impulses and links, and that we have moved into a new knowledge paradigm; one where we have started to believe in the power of quantum truth, of quantum transformation.

The study by Paul Bach-y-Rita was in response to a debilitating stroke from his father. Because of this, he was encouraged to practice brain therapy and began developing his father's cognitive brain activities that were so effective in restoring his mind-body relation that his father fully recovered. The husband of Bach-y-Rita went from being crippled to scaling the mountains! Eventually, the science community started listening and experimenting.

Barbara Arrowsmith began working with the creation of brain exercises in the 1980s to improve the function of her brain. She did this because she grew up with what was then described as a mental block, but was in fact a range of serious learning disabilities. She learned and wrote all backwards, had difficulty conceptualizing words, and was unable to grasp the interactions to the extent that she found it difficult to do anything like crossing the street. She was unable to feel discomfort in her body's left side and was getting badly injured all the time. The life of Barbara Arrowsmith was more than difficult until she found some research showing that her problem was related to a specific part of her brain. She decided she was going to fix it. She also developed techniques to relax and wake up her brain parts that have not performed so well. It's been bold... and it succeeded. Arrowsmith developed all kinds of brain exercises to boost her brain. She would do stuff like drawing clocks over and over again; rendering times distinct before her brain started tracking the clock's hand-to-hand interaction. She started seeing a massive improvement in the way her brain behaved in a matter of weeks. She was able to immerse herself in all sorts of interesting theoretical texts in a matter of months when she was initially unable to understand and conceptualize. In a way, she hadn't been able to understand before. Eventually, her imagination could make sense of things, so she transformed her life for the better.

The brain may be changing. It was built for transformation, reorganization and improvement; it's what it was born to do. Now that we understand the principles of quantum physics and start applying these concepts in order to heal ourselves, we are finding how remarkable these changes can be. Over 300 billion neurons and an almost infinite number of possible connections are in our brains. Our minds have more cells than stars in the sky. We have so much potential for change and development, and within autism we have so much potential for change and growth.

It's a rebellion. In almost every disorder you may think about, we will push the brain right, Add, OCD, Autism... brain plasticity will become the future's major player. Dr. Michael Merzenich, a world-famous neuroscientist,' meta-plasticity' is the latest thing in neuroplasticity. Because meta-cognition is a deeper understanding of your mind (Meta means' over,' cognition is thought), meta-plasticity is knowledge of the plasticity of your brain. This sounds great, but it actually means that people are thinking at how to get the brain more capable of being flexible, more capable of changing. We look at cognitive health, and the more the brain changes, the more it learns how to improve. The more it improves the better and better it gets. Every brain can change and improve. At change, each brain can get better and better. There's the chance of dynamic change inside autism. Anat Baniel (Kids beyond Limits author) and others are doing outstanding work with autists by helping them reconnect their brain and body. Gently helped them learn to master their body-mind connection, they learn to feel safe, secure and awake; they learn to let the world in. The plasticity of the brain has much to offer to the autist. The only thing to remember is that the organ must be included in brain plasticity. Kinesthetically, children learn. Kinesthetically, we all think. You know with your hands, you use your body to process information. Learning is sensitive and tactile. It's a natural, biological system to take new knowledge—it transforms you, it becomes part of you. We have the ability to retrain the minds, but it's important to remember that when we continue to include the body, we do this much more effectively, as all training takes place in the body.

Chapter 11 How To Implement This Argument on Health Care

How Does Polyvagal Treat Autism?

Autism is a neurodevelopment disorder. It usually emerges between the age of two and three years. An individual diagnosed with autism may experience challenges in social skills, language development, and repetitive behaviors. The disorder is usually more common to boys as compared to girls. Based on previous research, approximately one in eighteen children is diagnosed with the disorder.

Autism spectrum disorder is its full name. The name is based on the fact that an individual will experience mild, moderate, and severe symptoms. Lots of parents in the world do not want to spend the necessary time to learn all about this disorder. They live in a life of self-denial, arguing baselessly that the disease cannot happen to their children.

The disorder was first discovered in the 1930s. The causes of the dysfunction remain unknown to date. Once you have observed sure signs and symptoms from your child connected to the disorder, contact the services of a doctor, it is never too early for screening and evaluation. In fact, the earlier, the better. Nevertheless, it is not too late. An older child or an adult should also go for screening if symptoms are noted.

Currently, there are many effective treatments for the disorder, but there is no known cure. The procedures are mainly medical, which also includes therapies regarding speech, occupation, developmental, and behaviors. It is incomplete to talk about autism treatment without necessarily mentioning Polyvagal treatment.

According to professor Stephen Porges, autistic individuals are known to possess characters that trouble them in regulating their emotions and behaviors. Based on his research, neural regulation of the bodily organs influences emotional responses and behavioral responses toward other human beings and the environment. Many people with autism disorder are known not to respond positively to dangerous situations and environmental conditions. From the realization professor, Porges came up with The Polyvagal Theory, which explains more on the treatment of the disorder.

The theory explains more about three parts of the majorly used nervous system. This is the autonomic nervous system, the sympathetic nervous system, and the parasympathetic nervous system. From the name polyvagal, you can understand that it comes from the vagus nervous system.

The vagus nerves are usually paired but usually referred to in the singular. It originates from the medulla oblongata and supplies necessary nerve fibers to the esophagus, heart, lungs, intestinal tract, throat, and windpipe, and the colon's transverse portion. The theory helps us to understand that both branches of the vagus nerves help to calm down the body but in different ways. It is an explanation of how the vagus nerves work in the body to help control various body conditions. The nerve is enrolled with tasks that are vital for human survival.

Vagus nerve stimulation treats body condition by following a precise medical procedure by utilizing a device that triggers the nerve stimulating it to a specific stimulus. It can be done manually or by the use of electrical appliances. The effectiveness of the stimulation has been tested through several clinical tests and approved by the board of food and drug administration as a treatment for specific conditions.

People living with autism are known to perceive different conditions that can be solved or minimized by the use of polyvagal treatment. Some of the situations include;

Handling of Their Emotions

People with autism are generally regarded as lacking empathy and cannot understand emotions that are different from individuals without the condition. However, that notion is wrong, and they only perceive emotions differently from people without the state. In some cases, autistic people experience excessive feelings and empathy in different situations. In research, an autistic person confessed about his intense compassion to the death of his sister while other autistic volunteers agreed that the expression of emotions and empathy is complicated for them.

Based on Professor Stephen Porges' report, stimulation of the vagus nerve boosts an individual's memory, which triggers your emotions. Stimulation of the vagus nerve releases a special neurotransmitter, a substance referred to as norepinephrine, which collects in the amygdala, which consolidates the individual's memories and emotions. It is through the activation of the nerve that a person is able to perceive different emotions in the right manner. Polyvagal treatment of autism disorder is acknowledged by doctors as a method of treating and autistic people.

Neuroception

Have you ever been in a situation where you feel unsafe or uncertain? When in such conditions, the body through the central nervous system triggers the brain to take adequate measures to escape from the danger. People with autism spectrum disorder perceive dangerous situations in a different manner. In some cases, they perceive dangerous situations lightly, which keeps their lives on risks.

In Polyvagal theory, Doctor Porges describes the process in which the neural circuits are leading causes of danger in the environment known as neuroception. Through neuroception, people with autism experience the world in a way that they involuntarily scan situations and people to determine if they are safe or dangerous.

From the doctor, the vagus nerve determines the process of neuroception, which can be used to treat autism. This is through stimulation of the vagus nerve. In the process, both sides of the vagus nerve are stimulated. This is because both sides, usually the ventral and dorsal sides, are useful in determining how we perceive from our environment and social interactions. The ventral side, when stimulated, determines how we respond to cues of safety while the ventral side determines how we react to signals of danger. When autistic individual vagus nerves are stimulated, they become aware of the environments that they are in, and hence they respond appropriately.

Treatment of Epilepsy

Based on research, people with autism are at risk of being affected by epilepsy. Polyvagal treatment of epilepsy can be used to attend to the situation if it arises. This is through Vagus nerve stimulation. Epilepsy is characterized by frequent seizures, and this nerve technique reduces the frequency by which seizures occur and is mostly applicable in people who have complications with given medications. It is an add-on medical therapy, which means that it is utilized together with another medicine.

The simulator is programmed to generate impulses of electricity at regular intervals, depending on how much you can take. Do not attempt it on your own. The doctor will re-program it in the office. You are given a magnet that, when brought near to the stimulator, a direct current of low voltage electricity is generated that reduces the severity and the occurrence of the seizures.

Anxiety

Anxiety disorders are known to affect more than forty-two percent of people living with an autistic spectrum disorder. This is because they are not able to express how they feel in regard to different situations. Anxiety can trigger racing heart, muscle tightness while others feel frozen. It all depends on how the effectors translate and react to the stimuli. Every individual has a different way of response concerning the degree of the stimuli and depending on past experiences of the same or close stimuli. Some may even have a heart attack and succumb to death. However, it is rare, but there is a low probability of having such cases.

According to doctor Stephen's theory, anxiety is controlled by the vagus nerve operations. When the nerves are stimulated, the body responds by releasing hormone acetylcholine. From this stimulation, vagus nerve tendrils become active, extending its fiber-optic like cables connected to several body organs relaying information and instructions to release prolactin, enzymes, and protein, which help to relieve the anxiety. The Polyvagal Theory stipulates that stimulation of the vagus nerve in the body of an autistic person is an excellent tool to help ease his anxiety.

Stress Management

Stress is one of the significant barriers to a fulfilled life of a person living with an autism spectrum disorder. It cuts across the spectrum disorder at all stages of their lives. Stress affects everyone. However, autistic people are highly susceptible to high levels of unhealthy stress. Some of the notable symptoms of stress among autistic individuals include increased anxiety, highly irritable, losing temper, low esteem, and headaches.

Polyvagal theory by doctor Stephen Porges is a crucial tool that, when applied, can help to cope with stress. The doctor believed that stress is caused by an imbalance of neurotransmitter hormones. This can be solved by stimulation of the vagus nerve. When the nerve is stimulated, the brain responds by releasing hormone neurotransmitters to body organs, which help to relieve the stress. This is an important technique that can be used to help individuals living with the disorder.

Living with a person with an autistic spectrum disorder has its challenges. It is also a situation that many families are going through. There are many things that you can do to help people with the disorder. Being emotionally stable is a necessity to live with individuals.

Accept them as they are- rather than focusing much on how autistic individuals are different, it's always right to try and identify what they are lacking. Accept all their quirks and celebrate their success regardless of how minor they are.

Try and learn about autism- the more you know about the disorder, the more you become aware of how you can handle autistic people. You are able to make informed decisions regarding how you treat the individuals. Educate yourself more about treatment options, and always ensure that you participate in all treatment decisions.

What Is Sensory Processing Disorder?

At times, an individual may produce abnormal or different response compared to the information perceived. This happens if the individual is having a neurological disorder referred to as sensory integration dysfunction or famously used term sensory processing disorder.

In plain English, it means that your child's senses—smell, sight, taste, touch, sound, and proprioception (the 6th sense)—are either overactive or underactive. When something engages their senses, they do not respond to the trigger in a "normal" way.

This can manifest in different ways and across multiple senses at once. It ranges from severe and debilitating to mild, to the point no one understands there is a sensory problem.

Chapter 12 Taking Action Against Anxiety

Action Plan To Follow for Fighting Anxiety and Panic Attacks

Countless people suffer from anxiety every day. Some have brief periods when anxiety renders them incapable of carrying out a task and think rationally about the situation. At other times, anxiety can appear without warning while going through your routine. Two people who experience anxiety cannot relate exactly to each other.

Anxiety is often brought on by emotionally charged situations and stress-inducing circumstances. If you have gone through the process of acknowledging your anxiety, and now you want to take charge of the situation, you must know that it is not an easy task. It is an uphill battle. Saying that with perseverance and determination, you can overcome anxiety and lead a happy and prosperous life.

Some medications and therapies will help you set along to the path for recovery, but in the end, it is up to you to take the reins of your own recovery. It is up to you to find and adhere to practices that will bring about positivity and productivity in your life that anxiety tends to purge away from you regularly. So these are some of the things you can practice to mitigate anxiety from your life.

Whenever anxiety starts to loom, you will start to get negative thoughts. It will constantly remind you of your failures. So a good practice to break free from this and halt anxiety right in its tracks is to take a step back and acknowledge all the positive things that are around you. It is not all gloom and doom as your nervousness was making you believe. If you experience negativity in certain situations because of your anxiety, then it helps to look at the possible positives of the situation.

Writing down can help you with your experiences with anxiety. Journaling your thoughts is a very positive coping mechanism. It not only helps you get it out of your system, but when you are in a more peaceful state, you can reflect on the emotions and thoughts that stormed over you. You can logically deal with anxiety.

Organize and set up a routine for your life. It will help you avoid cluttering, which brings about unnecessary stress and panic.

Practice the techniques that your therapist has suggested. Whatever they may be, meditation, breathing or spending time outdoors. Make room in your life for them.

Practice healthy eating and exercise.

Don't berate yourself on feeling anxiety; it is normal. There are some grounding techniques you can learn to avoid panic and anxiety. There are also breathing exercises you can turn to whenever you feel a panic attack approaching. Worrying about future events will not make them right.

Try and will yourself to have a healthier perspective in life. There is always light at the end of the tunnel.

Don't ignore or neglect your anxiety. Try to acknowledge and learn awareness about it.

Here are some simple tips to avoid anxious thoughts that bring on anxiety and panic attacks.

1. Your mind is not hardwired to deal with things in a certain way from a young age. We do feel like that because we often find ourselves reacting to things the same way our parents tend to do. You should know it is not the case. You don't have to do things the way your parents do if it's causing harm. You can consciously change and be flexible about your approach to circumstances.

2. We tend to overthink things, and without even realizing it, we are reacting to it and making it very personal. This is a very negative habit. You have to learn which things should matter. You choose the things that affect you. For an anxious person, you have to develop awareness to deal with your thoughts objectively.

3. You have to learn to let go of things and not let every other comment that others say get to you. It can cause a lot of problems for your mental health.

4. Getting close to yourself is a sure way to beat anxiety as it often stems from the insecurity you feel in the first place.

5. Observe yourself, your thoughts, and your emotions. Bring yourself at peace with your thoughts. Take a moment to relish in the state of calmness. Remind yourself that this is what your true nature is. You are not your scattered thoughts and anxiety. You will eventually like this side of you and consciously make an effort to get on the track to your true nature.

6. It also helps to keep the present moment as a sort of anchor to elude anxiety and panic. Taking a step back and observing the situation really helps with the stress that threatens to upstage your peace of mind. Practice open-mindedness and accept situations to move on from them, rather than carrying their emotional baggage for the future.

Getting Rid of Anxiety

Here are some of the things that can help ward off anxiety daily.

- Exercise daily.

- Incorporate meditation in your daily life.

- Cleaning could take your mind off of worrying.

- Try to spend time in nature.

- Humans are social creatures. Try to spend time in the good company of your friends.

- Aromatherapy is an amazing way to lower your stress level.

- Uncertainty about your future often causes anxiety. It helps to pen down your goals and look forward to taking steps to realize them.

- Eat plenty of healthy stuff and drink an appropriate amount of water.

- There is nothing worse than what not getting enough sleep could do for your mental health. Sleep deprivation hyper-activates the areas of the brain related to emotional processing and sets of neural activity that imitates anxiety. (Ph.D., 2019)

- Take supplements to regulate the amount of iron and vitamin B in your body. They are responsible for regulating serotonin in your body.

- Chamomile tea is a great stress diffuser.

- Instead of watching shows that put you on edge, try picking up light-hearted and funny shows that make you see the lighter side of life.

- Recently, coloring has been coming up as a great stress reliever, and people say it makes their symptoms fade away.

When you feel a panic attack approaching, you can practice these two very useful ways to deal with it.

- Relax your muscles. Start from one end of your body and finish at another. You can tense up one group of muscle at a time for a few moments and then release it after some more seconds.

- Just try to acknowledge the symptoms that a panic attack brings about. Don't try to fight them, but tell yourself these are normal panic symptoms and are brought about because my mind is causing them. Just stay with your panic attacks instead of neglecting and being stubborn about accepting it.

Chapter 13 How To Meditate

You must have had an awful time in your life where you felt bad. Such feelings and emotions occur when one is apprehensive or traumatic. In psychology, there is a terminology used, which is a meditation that encompasses reaching ultimate conscience. Introspection has been a technique of reaching to a peaceful mind. It is mainly used by individuals participating in Yoga or mindfulness. People may ask where meditation and mindfulness relate. First of all, mindfulness is pondering to capture your inner feelings and trying to understand your present emotions. In other words, you are trying to feel the moment.

Therefore, mindfulness-mediation is the exercise of concentrating on your conscience without thinking on the past or future. This practice involves also breathing simulation, mental visualization, awareness of the environment, and muscle and body relaxation. Since this activity is not judgmental, its primary purpose is accomplishing a good state of mind and relieving any stress or anxiety. Having a peaceful mental state ensures you focus on the issues relating to benefitting your life.

How Mindfulness Works

This program aims to bring our brain at maximum concentration when capturing the feeling of the environment. Therefore. It is advisable to be alone when undertaking the procedure. That means minimal interruptions and disturbance.

However, to carry such a process successfully one has to consider the following steps of successful mindfulness mediation.

The first step is the preparation stage or the preliminary action. This aspect involves choosing the best sites to ruminate, like at your house balcony or river stream. Think of the posture you are going to sit and relax because this particular program requires comfortability. Carry a manual guide that directs you on the operation. Lastly, prepare your mind and relieve any emotions that can hinder you from thinking appropriately.

Take a deep puff of air and relax. Have a large gulp of air and commensurate on your breathing rhythm. This activity will help one to release any fatigue of the brain hence making you think straightforward about the present situation. Reflect of the reverberations around you and try to apprehend their pitch. Enjoy the feeling of that sound and recapture every moment like of the birds tweeting and chirping. Finally, keep taking and releasing slow and deep breaths until you feel relaxed.

The next step is to close your eyes. This activity helps one to concentrate on their thoughts fully. This action helps to reflect on what you want your life to be. Try to forget the bad things happening to you and prioritize on the right stuff. Think of how sweet your life has been and how preciously you want to be successful. Let your dreams be the first thoughts that come in.

Again, focus on your breath as a whole. Conceptualize at your breathing rate and rhythm. Feel the freshness and the aroma of the air. Contemplate on how the cold air gets inside and how the hot breadth comes outside. Picture the chest rising and how the ribs shrink. Master, all your inhalation activities as this, will help you open your mind and improve your focus. Let this operation be natural, and do not control your inhalation rate at any moment. Lastly, be mindful about the breathing patterns you can count one up to ten and start the game again. Soon you will realize that this method is working for you appropriately.

After trying that procedure, if your thoughts are still not definite, repeat the process this time around getting more absorbed to the inspiration rate. Twitch to realize the capacity, rapidity, temperateness, and how that air travels through the windpipe and into the lungs. Master every chest opening and closing at every inhalation interval. Once the brain settles reflect on your consciousness fully alongside the rhythmic breathing.

At this stage, you should bring your thoughtfulness to the contemplations that flow. Try to take them from the inspiration and notice every thought, in that case, master it and analyze those feelings. You will be surprised at the level of how the thoughts stream your mind. Do not get carried away by the happiness of realizing the brain inflows, but let them travel to through the sensor.

The last step is the reflection phase. At this moment, you have already thought enough; therefore create a visual or imagery reflection upon what you are sensitizing. Experience a mounting sense of tranquility inside you and center for more concentration. One warning is that do not let the emotions get the better part of you because they are a disruption. That should not be the point where you start crying, being anxious, or overjoyed.

Mindfulness for Stress and Anxiety Reduction

Stress and anxiety make us not to think straight. Anxiety and stress even make you anticipate less useful things. The state of being anxious means, the mind is not at rest and is pressurized to commit to planned action. Imagine how you behaved, when you were a kid when your folks informed you that you would go for a trip, did you sleep that night? Indeed, you did not because you were eager to go for that trip. Stress, in other words, is a load of thinking in one's brain that cannot be solved at an instance.

How Can One Calm Such Feelings?

The practice helps one to explore the underlying causes of your pressures. When in mindfulness, the brain is relaxed, and one can remember even a solution to a problem. It is also evident that when a mind is fresh, its creativity rate is high. Therefore, one can efficiently innovate a way to curb stress. Gaining insight into your troubles enables one to structure them into a workable formula.

The program helps in creating a space for your worries. Sometimes one is pressured because you are not thinking of a problem correctly. It may result from the mental area of those feelings. When undertaking this therapy, it helps in releasing the junk in mind. You may be astonished that after going through the treatment, solutions of particular problems start arising.

Always be intentional. There is where you put all your objectives before anything else. Having stress or anxiety is a degradation to your commitments and goals. Have an insight into what to see you in the future. When one thinks about that during a mindful stage, it overshadows the bad feelings one possesses. This emotion helps you to develop tolerance in seeing yourself successful and valuable.

Act like a beginner. If it were possible, one would brain drain his mind to remove the pressurized piece. However, this is not possible even though one can program their cerebral to start thinking at a different angle. Always be free to adopt to ruminate issues at a different perspective, and by that, new opportunities can arise. These possibilities can help you fight any anxiety, feelings, and thoughts.

Mindful behavior is nonjudgmental. Therefore, one cannot process the bad feelings they had before. That is a way of filtering the bad from the good. Hey, try to judge the stress in another perspective like, it is not a problem but a challenge or platform to push you to opportunities. When you have such a mindset, it enables one to view stress as an advantage. When you stop judgmental protocols, many anxiety moods go away.

Where To Practice Mindfulness

Mindfulness can be practiced in the body. The body is an expression to the nature and the response to the physical movement of a being. It contains all organs that are pivotal to human living. The body shapes the appearance of a person where these features nurture how other people perceive. For example, some people view short people as weak and tall people as brave. Mindfulness is used to help one appreciate the change of appearance, which somebody should accept. Especially for people greeting old they should understand that and not feel lousy during the mindfulness session. For that reason, mindfulness is preparation for the body of what can happen.

This aspect is used in controlling our emotions, moods, and attitudes. Some people are fearful of doing something like an activity. Being allergic to something is sometimes your mindset, and only careful meditation can help to remove such a weird notion. Our thoughts, our minds, and our actions make feelings of what we do.

Application to a state of mind is another example. Those who have mental issues like stress and anxiety it means their state of mind is somehow corrupted. Some other people are intoxicated after indulging in drugs hence changing their state of mind. There are other times you feel tired and assumes to rest because' you are not thinking clearly.' When undergoing mindfulness, you refresh your brains and forget about your problems or fatigues. It also helps one's mind to be relaxed just like sleeping.

Application to medicine. This activity has a medicinal value where people are advised to carry out the procedure. When you focus on cognition, it means you use your fat levels appropriately; therefore, disease lie diabetes, obesity, and other ones are reduced. It also brings happiness. Consequently, you cannot suffer from depression, ulcers, and additional stress-related disorders.

It is easy to learn this method of meditation because it is straightforward. All you need to do is to find a quiet and comfortable space and put aside troubling thoughts. Mindfulness meditation is readily available to us any time we want to practice it. You can also incorporate mindfulness meditation in your life when doing household activities. There's no specific rule for doing mindfulness meditation. You can meditate when washing dishes. Have you realized how no one bothers you when you are washing the dishes? This is the perfect opportunity to practice mindfulness meditation and let go of disturbing thoughts. The water and the bubbles in the sick create a serene environment for meditation. When you let go and enjoy the experience, your mind is refreshed, and you find inner peace.

Another chance to meditate is when you are brushing your teeth. You brush your teeth every day, so there is no excuse not to meditate. Feel the brush you are holding, your feet firmly on the ground, and practice mindfulness meditation. You can also meditate when driving or during exercise. You can exercise 10 minutes in the morning as you practice mindfulness meditation. Watching television while exercise makes you finish quickly, but you benefit more when you include mindfulness meditation. Furthermore, you can meditate at bedtime by enjoying the thoughts instead of rushing through them. You will feel more relaxed and sleep soundly. Spend time with your children before you put them to bed. Listen to them, look into their eyes, and take in every moment.

Chapter 14 How Others Manage To Have Strong Confidence

You might be having someone in your mind who you think is overconfident. I am sure that you might be asking yourself how they manage to be such confident. According to research, most confident people have used a lot of time to build up their confidence, so it does not happen overnight.

A survey done to over 500 exceptionally confident executives shows that they used a combination of tactics to become confident. No one would have to be confident in life so as to pursue their goals and good speakers and performers. You might be wondering about where to start. The following are the ways in which other people managed to have a strong self-confident.

They Have Role Models

Confident people choose role models to emulate, and they pick up their qualities. They also develop those qualities for themselves to become confident. You can apply this trick Into Your Life by finding a role model.

They Have Connections

Confident people have a strong network and useful contact. These people will allow them to keep connections for ideas sharing and upgrading their careers. You should also find a network or upgrade your network to benefit from strong self-confidence.

They Do Not Give in to the Self-Doubt

Those people who seem to be confidence realize that they are in a position of leadership, and they cannot afford to give in to their self-doubt. You should also realize your role and work hard towards achieving your goals.

They Prioritize

They have accepted the fact that they have lots of things to do and cannot do all at the same time. You should also realize that you need to first take care of your priorities.

They Are Kind to Themselves

Taking the first priority on yourself is the first thing that you should do. It is all about you; take care of yourself first so that you will be able to deliver your best.

Secrets Confident People Don't Want You To Know About Speaking on Stage

There is nothing complicated that confident people do while speaking on stage. It is all about mastering the tips that we have learned previously. You might admire your favorite speaker because of the way they manage to capture people's attention and get them hooked all the way and you are left wondering whether you can be like them.

They can combine entertaining, teaching, and some fun. When these people are addressing, you cannot look away, you will not get bored, and you will process all the teaching that they gave.

The following are 4 simple secrets that they apply.

Secret #1: They Convey Emotions

Courageous public speakers and performers apply emotions in their presentations. Conveying emotions to your audience through the tone of your voice or your body language is very important in conveying your message. SO, think hard about the emotions you would like your audiences to feel.

Secret #2: They Apply Leadership Mindset

Another secret is to realize that the audience sees a presenter as a leader with a certain authority. After realizing this, they are able to apply the expectations of their audience. You can also apply his secrets in your next presentation; do as a leader would do.

Secret #3 They Make Good Use of Body Language

Successful public speakers and presenters understand how to assign the various meaning of their body language. They know how to move, gesture, stand, or deal with nervousness. For you to be at the exact same level, you need to do a bit of practice; you can rehearse applying various body languages before your next presentation.

Secret #4 Pay Attention to the Vocal Tone

Another secret to a successful presentation is to make good use of your vocal tone. Successful presenters and speakers have mastered this tactic and use it to convey their message effectively. The volume of your voice, articulations, modulation, or well-placed pauses is very powerful for an effective presentation.

Mental Block on Stage? Here Is the Solution

Mental block causes stage fright. A mental block occurs when you are in the center stage ready to give a presentation, and all over sudden, no words come out of your mouth.

Mental block on stage can occur even if you had a thorough prior preparation. There are various reasons why mental block on stage occurs. One of the main reasons for this is the lack of strong self-confidence. Fear of rejection and humiliation by the audience is also another main reason why most people experience mental block.

Mental block on stage can sometimes be embarrassing, but the good thing is that there are ways to overcome these mental blocks. These include:

1. Practice Thoroughly

Practice makes perfect, but it also acts as a brain trainer. It helps inject into your subconscious mind everything that you have planned to say. When your brain is highly trained, it will easily be able to recall all the necessary points.

2. Get Used to Public Performance

When practicing, you don't have to practice on your own. You can gather a small crowd such as your friends or your workmates. These will help you to get read of fears slowly and build up confidence for the actual presentation or performance

3. Avoid Perfectionist Mind

When your mind is looking to do perfect work, this will be hard for yourself and could contribute to a mental block. It is important for you to relax and accept the fact that it is fine to make mistakes.

4. Take a Deep Breath

Some things will make you feel nervous on stage, such as when you make a mistake. This could lead to a mental block, but you can manage it by taking time to pause and take a deep breath so as you will gain your momentum.

5. Get Enough Sleep the Night Before Your Performance

Make sure that you relax and sleep well the night before the presentation. This will make your body to refresh and activate the brain's power for it to function well.

Beating the mental block is a simple thing to do. You just need to pay attention to that thing that causes the mental block. Using the above simple tips, you will be able to gain self-confidence and perform well on stage.

Chapter 15 A Better Life

Clearly, some anxiety is normal but too much can lead to major problems including PTSD. Remember, if you need help, simply ask for it. To my knowledge, a life without worry, which is perfect, does not exist. Nevertheless, we know that there is relief from worry and hope for the future - Because of the many ways we can care for ourselves. Just as there are individuals with compassionate hearts, we can have compassion for ourselves. We can also change a stressful way of life to one that exterminates or diminishes anxiety; as a reminder, this is how:

Diminish or do not use drugs such as caffeine and alcohol

Pinpoint what makes you stressed and eliminate or reduce the causes of stress

Replace your unhealthy ways of coping with healthy ways

Enrich your relationships by communicating assertively and compassionately

Use time management so that you feel in control of your life

Follow a nutritious daily diet (use a variety of whole rather than refined foods)

Hydrate yourself well by drinking plenty of fresh water

Have regular meal times

Eat within a nice environment

Do breathing, relaxation and movement activities daily

Have good-enough sleep patterns

Design a healthy life-style, as personal needs and wants change

All of these factors ease anxiety away while sweetening the life we live.

As for PTSD specifically, there is a relatively recent (early 21st century) therapeutic technique, called 'rewind', for which robust research is needed to ascertain whether it works sufficiently enough for most people, but currently, there is some clinical evidence that it does work for some, as in the case of Zoe, below.

Start of case study

Zoe suffered from sleeplessness, bad dreams and repeated flashbacks about several attacks that happened to her over a period of several years, before she was old enough to leave her parental home. Just like a vast number of families (perhaps most if not practically all), hers was dysfunctional. Yet, she did not want to disclose certain details about what she went through in her home of origin.

One day, she found out that a therapist not far from where she worked used a technique for PTSD, where the client did not have to reveal any details. At the first meeting with that therapist, he made sure that Zoe was in a fully and deeply relaxed state. He enabled her to imagine being in a place where she felt completely at ease and utterly safe. Then, she was encouraged to bring her anxiety to the fore and he again encouraged her to experience being in that safe place so she became at ease once more.

When this was achieved, he talked Zoe into an even deeper state of relaxation. While in that relaxed state, the therapist asked her to imagine being at her safe place where there was a television set and DVD player with remote control. Next, he told her to imagine floating out of her body and sitting to one side of her physical body so that she could watch the Zoe that floated out of her, look at the TV screen, without watching the screen herself. In this way, she watched a 'film' of whatever the traumatic event or situations were to the point where there was no more trauma and she re-experienced feeling safe.

After this, the therapist asked Zoe to imagine floating back into her body and feel herself going very quickly backwards via the trauma from the safe place to the safe place; as if she was an image on a DVD film that was being re-wound.

When that was achieved, her asked her to imagine watching the same images as if they were on the TV, which she pressed the fast-forward button on the remote control.

All of these aspects were repeated many times, backwards and forwards, at the speed that Zoe was comfortable with, until none of the scenes had any emotional reaction from her.

Since Zoe was still afraid of being with her family of origin, and there was a likelihood that this would occur at a funeral, while she was in a relaxed state, the therapist told her to see herself as a confident and assertive woman with the family. She successfully did as he said. That is when her therapy finished.

End of case study

'Rewind' must only be conducted by a person who is trained, qualified and experienced with doing it. This is because of the risk of an inexperienced person re-traumatising the sufferer. So do not try it on your own. You can help yourself by first learning and understanding 'rewind' in a highly skilled way, if it is something you would like to experience.

Case studies I have presented have used evidence-based strategies for healing. There is a different type of evidential base other than empirical. I am talking about clinical evidence. Indeed, from my own personal experience, what I have found extremely useful is being with a person that I feel safe with, and learning how to calm down by relaxing using the methods I have described in this book. Also beneficial are experiencing forms of art that bring out my positive emotions, such as watching a funny film that makes me laugh out loud, viewing a beautiful painting and personally doing some arty-crafty activities, as well as listening to melodic Disney songs, playing a musical instrument, and dancing. The aroma of sweet-smelling flowers, the taste of juicy fresh fruit and stroking a baby also work well for me. Using my facial muscles, breathing in a way that calms me down and moving in different ways using all the muscles in my body, as well as being with another that I can have a relatively good relationship with, all connect with my heart, and boost me for the better. All these things increase heart regulation for me. I am not alone. This happens to others too! For example, if we are in a friendly relationship, we feel good and this shifts our physiological state in a healthy way.

Be informed by your own experiences! Opening our hearts with compassion for self and others, no matter who they are, is basic, sounds simple and is amazingly healing. Remember to think of what makes you feel good, allow that emotion into your heart and expand how you feel, while breathing calmly with an open mind. Let self-compassion overflow to others, relax, be at ease with yourself, no matter what. When in this state, it is impossible to have a PTSD symptom; so my strong suggestion is: do it daily for half an hour each time. Do not fall into the trap of making excuses such as 'I have problems because I come from a dysfunctional family'. I have yet to meet a person whose family of origin was not dysfunctional. Do not let this stop you from social activities.

We are born, to be socially engaged. It is one of the reasons why babies like playing peek-a-boo. There is a feeling of safety engendered during non-aggressive play. Playing with machines such as i-pads is not better than playing directly person-to-person. Just remember that personal hygiene is important therefore have a good wash every day, so you do not have a distasteful smell when meeting another. For myself, I like a cool shower after a warm bath; doing so suspends any stressful thoughts I might have. A belief system that protects us fearfully stops humane development because of the defensive type of protection. It also limits creativity and buffers against feeling safe. We all need to feel safe and when we do, our fearless humaneness expands while developing solutions and creativity flourishes. Let go of fear. That is the challenge. Our health depends so very much on our feelings.

For sure, the emotions we feel change the way we think, have an effect on our actions, and impact on our overall health; depending on what feelings are in our hearts, this can be disastrous or can lead to an improved quality of life. Those of us, who have worked through this book, experienced for ourselves how to change the emotions we feel so that our thoughts are more helpful to us, consequently changing our behaviour, resulting in not only busting any excessive worrying and PTSD but also in improving our general wellness. These are very useful skills for creating a better life. I hope you will pass on each skill you have learnt, to others who can benefit from them.

Chapter 16 Autism Spectrum Disorders

The term autism spectrum disorders (ASD) incorporates autism, Asperger's disorder, and different conditions. (ADHD isn't characterized as an autism spectrum disorder.) ASD includes a wide scope of side effects, levels of debilitation, and incapacities that can show up in kids or grown-ups. These manifestations, thought to be formative cerebrum disorders, can cause critical social, conduct, and correspondence challenges. In any case, there are no neural tests for these disorders.

There are various classes of autism. The disorders influence every individual in an extraordinary manner and range from extremely gentle to serious. Individuals with autism spectrum disorders share a portion of similar side effects and appear to deal with data in their cerebrum uniquely in contrast to other individuals do. The precise reasons for autism spectrum disorders are obscure. Research proposes that the two qualities and condition assume significant jobs. The proof indicating qualities is situated partially on the perception that in the event that one indistinguishable twin is mentally unbalanced, there is a decent possibility that the other twin will be also. Be that as it may, regardless of burning through a huge number of dollars, scientists still can't seem to distinguish which qualities might be damaged in instances of autism. In a perfect world, this will be resolved soon; however, at present, there is no encouraging remedy for autism spectrum disorder dependent on hereditary research.

Autism-spectrum conclusions depend fundamentally on clinicians' perceptions of conduct. Be that as it may, the individuals doing the testing don't normally consider the physiological indications of the social-commitment bit of the autonomic nervous system. In any case, the autonomic nervous system, to some degree, decides the emotional state, and the emotional state is a contributing variable in deciding conduct.

May a few instances of autism spectrum disorder be comprehended as appearances of autonomic nervous system disorder? These people are regularly in a ceaseless state of either battle or-flight or dorsal vagal withdrawal. Once in a while, for no apparent reason, they move all of a sudden, starting with one of these states then onto the next, finding overseers napping. Their conduct is as often as possible eccentric and wrong for the circumstance.

It is prescribed that autism-spectrum tests ought to incorporate assessment of the capacity of their ventral vagus nerve. On the off chance that it shows brokenness, further research could tell in the case of bringing the patient into a state of social commitment by improving the capacity of this nerve achieves positive changes in their conduct. It is my conviction this would be the situation.

Autism and the Autonomic Nervous System

Activity of the spinal sympathetic chain, or potentially dorsal vagal activity, can be physiological qualities of the nervous system of individuals with different conclusions on the autism spectrum. They may likewise have a physical issue emerging from a brokenness in their organs.

Their family or parental figures may see that individuals with autism some of the time respond with dread and frenzy even with no apparent reason. They might be easily affected, responding to an improvement in the condition that other individuals don't see, or to something that helps them to remember something from quite a while ago—or they may just envision something perilous. Other individuals taking a gander at their conduct impartially find that these responses are unwarranted and feel there is not something to be disturbed about.

Once in a while, people on the autism spectrum are caught in states of battle or flight or shutdown or move between these two states. They might be in a state of shutdown, collapsed into themselves and emotionless one minute, at that point abruptly outgoing, apprehensive, or forceful in the following. To other people who don't comprehend their conduct, they respond in apparently bizarre, capricious ways that frequently cause them to appear to be asocial in their conduct. Numerous guardians or parental figures are confounded and shocked by these abrupt moves in conduct since they don't know about whatever could be causing the emotional changes. Mental testing for autism assesses conduct and characterizes various types of autism, however, doesn't think about the fundamental physiological factors regarding Porges' new elucidation of the capacity of the autonomic nervous system. Therefore, medications have, for the most part, centered around preparing the guardians to attempt to adjust their conduct to fit the extraordinary needs of their kid, as opposed to improving the kid's condition with the goal that they don't have these unique needs.

The Polyvagal Theory exhibits another bio-conduct model connecting medically introverted conduct to explicit physiological states of the autonomic nervous system. This permits us the likelihood to grow increasingly compelling methodologies for treating autism. At the point when we see that a large number of these people are being influenced by their spinal sympathetic chain or dorsal vagal activity, or are swaying between the two, we can basically say that they are not socially engaged. At that point, we can concentrate on utilizing or creating intercessions that help them to be socially engaged and improve the capacity of the ventral part of their vagus nerve and the other four related cranial nerves—bringing about progressively social practices.

Stephen Porges worked with mentally unbalanced kids and has had achievement in improving the conduct of huge numbers of them. He deciphered this as a check that there was some legitimacy to the model of the nervous system displayed in the Polyvagal Theory.

Treating Autism

Numerous such children have issues with typical social conduct; they don't appear to be keen on other individuals, abstaining from taking a gander at them or looking. They appear to need compassion and would prefer to invest energy alone or playing on their electronic gadgets. Their folks may assign other youngsters as "companions" in the event that they can sit together in a similar space for timeframes. In any case, the children don't generally associate with these companions, however, sit in their own universes, playing nearby one another yet without anyone else's input.

Some medically introverted people need verbal, relational abilities, and can-not partake in an important two-manner discussion. They don't appear to be ready to tune in or comprehend what is being stated, and they are not perky. Some don't speak by any means; others, when they do speak, may rehash like a parrot what was simply said by another person, or rehash sentences from a film. Some of the time they keep speaking without stopping for the other individual to react.

The sternocleidomastoid muscle is connected to the base of the temporal bone on the skull, so chronic tension in the SCM muscle perceptibly twists the shape of the skull with a specific goal in mind. Could certain trademark shapes of the skull put pressure on certain veins or nerves inside the skull? A baby's cranium is comprised of a few plates associated by extreme connective tissue. A consistent draw on the temporal bone from chronic tension in the SCM muscle can haul the baby's cranium rusty. On the off chance that the tension in the muscle isn't discharged, the skull stays flabby as the youngster develops.

Considerations in Treating Autistic Children
Treating children (particularly those on the autism spectrum) with hands-on procedures has its exceptional difficulties. Indeed, even children without autism will, for the most part, not lie still on a massage table for extremely long. Those with medicinal narratives have frequently had a background marked by endless visits to specialists and emergency clinics, where they have been compelled to lie still for an assessment, or to get excruciating infusions. It is difficult to envision how a kid with negative encounters like that can feel safe, particularly on the principal treatment—lying on her in a place of absolute weakness, in a new room, and being drawn nearer by a total more abnormal who towers over her and starts planning something for her. Obstruction is naturally activated by this, and it takes persistence, ability, and experience with respect to the advisor to enable these children to feel safe.

In the event that you are treating autistic children, there are a couple of things that you should know. At the point when they come into your space just because it is normal for them to feel unsafe. They don't have any acquaintance with you, and they frequently respond with dread after observing the massage table, which resembles a medicinal assessment table. You may have the best of helpful expectations. However, they don't have the foggiest idea about that. In the event that you or their folks hold them down, it is counterproductive; they will feel significantly increasingly undermined, and maybe disregarded.

A cardinal rule in treating children, particularly autistic children, is that they should feel safe, and must be regarded, consistently. This is an essential to specific strategies specifically that help the youngster's sensory system. One issue for autistic people who need ordinary two-way verbal correspondence is that they can't comprehend the expressed word alright to realize what's in store in a restorative experience. While the estimation of the treatment might be clear to their folks or to social insurance experts, autistic children may have no comprehension of why they are there or the worth they may pick up from the treatment. They no doubt have no clue that there is in any event, anything amiss with them, or that their life can be better. Their conduct changes, notwithstanding when they understand that they are safe with you, particularly once your treatment makes them feel better.

A typical trait of individuals on the autistic spectrum is that they experience issues conveying ordinarily, with individuals in their regular daily existence, yet in addition with their parental figures and with individuals attempting to treat them. These correspondence challenges limit the potential outcomes in their lives, just as the endeavors of others to speak with them and to treat them. This causes languishing over them and their families. Justifiably, their parental figures regularly feel powerless, tested, and not capable. Helping people on the autistic spectrum is an adventure into a huge, strange territory.

For parental figures and specialists, attempting to get a handle on the eccentricities of conduct showed by those on the autism spectrum may just add to the disarray. In any case, when we watch autistic people from the perspective of the Polyvagal Theory, we understand that we might have the option to help by basically improving the individual's ventral vagal capacity.

At some random minute, an individual can be in just one of the three autonomic states. Autism-spectrum people can all of a sudden move between conditions of pressure and withdrawal without others getting why. Empowering the condition of social engagement by improving the capacity of cranial nerves may can possibly balance out these movements and diminish a portion of the trouble that these people usually understanding. Besides, redressing sound-related issues by improving the capacity of the fifth and seventh cranial nerves frequently prompts emotional improvement in an individual's relational abilities, social practices, and compassion. Constructive changes of this nature will, in general, expand on themselves, further supporting the individual's improvement.

At the point when two individuals are socially engaged and imparting up close and personal, they pass data about their enthusiastic states by little developments of facial muscles. This additionally invigorates the nerves in the muscles of every individual's very own face, so their fifth and seventh cranial nerves give them continuous criticism and a reasonable thought of what they are feeling themselves and what they feel about the other individual. Our general public progressively depends on messages and instant messages. Television grapples regularly have dull faces, or expect put-on demeanors. An ever increasing number of individuals stifle their appearances with Botox or diminish their expressiveness with plastic medical procedure. Be that as it may, the more we convey without seeing every others' appearances and hearing the progressions of tone in one another's voices, the more indifferent the exchange will be, and the less we can impart anything inwardly. We can talk, yet with words alone, we are simply passing information.

Phones are a stage up in correspondence from messages since they catch changes in vocal articulation. Skype and FaceTime give us both the sound of the voice and the outward appearances —however, nothing beats up close and personal correspondence. The less children identify with grown-ups who impart completely utilizing a melodic voice and an expressive face, the more the children's facial expressivity will be underused and immature. Is anyone shocked that we have expanding quantities of children with autism, ADHD, and other correspondence issue?

Past identifying with autistic individuals, comparable troubles emerge now and again, identifying with any other person in any of our "typical" connections. Our associations with other individuals would be so natural if both we and they could be socially engaged constantly. Initially, it is useful to understand that we are not in a ventral vagal express constantly—nor are they. Second, we currently realize that we can plan something for bring ourselves or the other individual into a condition of social engagement.

It is my feeling that we have quite recently started to investigate the capability of the Polyvagal Theory not exclusively to help individuals on the autism spectrum however, to help every one of us in the entirety of our associations with others.

Concluding Remarks

While the Polyvagal Theory has given expanded clearness and comprehension with respect to treating different troublesome enthusiastic, physical, and states of mind, the experiences I've picked up into treatment of people on the autism spectrum have conceivably been the most significant.

Chapter 17 Time Management

Managing your time may not be on your list of priorities when consumed by worry that incorporates a phobia, and an uncomplicated option might be to be so busy, with busy-ness, that you say you have 'no time' for anything else. Work can take up much of our waking time. Yet, you can become extremely tired due to overworking, leading to an inability to fall asleep. Easy as it is in a civilisation of, continue-going-to-work-and-keep-working, do not allow yourself to be sucked into such an unhealthy culture for your good-health's sake. Instead, prioritise time-management so that you live a balanced life of play, labour and rest. Sometimes, waking when it feels as if everyone else the world sleeps is an inevitable self-sacrifice. For example, it may be necessary to do this for a period in life when having to breast-feed each night every two to three hours. However, this is normal and you know that baby will outgrow feeding at night. Therefore, there is no clinical problem. A good idea is to use your time between feeding, for sleeping yourself.

If there is little money coming into your household, you may be working in more than one place and very long hours, resulting in lack of sleep. You might be going 'the extra mile' with your work-hours because your pay is too low to not work more hours than most people. This, too, does not mean that you have a sleep problem. The issue here is financial. To deal with such a situation you can ask for a pay-rise in a non-apologetic, non-bullying way; you can ask in an assertive way. There are several assertiveness training courses on offer. There is a section on being assertive, further down. As for time management, have a go at worksheet 19 after copying it into your journal.

Start of worksheet 19

managing time worksheet

(follow the instructions)

Make daily, uninterrupted time for the following (I can do so by waking a few minutes earlier each day).

1. Understand my thought and behaviour patterns

2. Relax

3. While relaxing, create my goal of what I want

4. Stay relaxed while adding emotion to my vision

5. See my goal mentally as clearly as possible, as if I have it now

6. Make a plan of putting it into action and do something daily towards that (write in my diary what I will do daily so that I allocate time for it)

7. Adjust my life appropriately (for instance, if I take up time for putting vision into action, then let go of what I would have done during that time)

8. Connect with like-minded individuals (schedule this into my diary)

End of worksheet 19

Putting vision into action works even if you think 'I've too much to do', or 'I don't have time' (assuming you incorporate number '7' in the worksheet immediately above). You can expect results within a month of doing everything in worksheet 19, daily for ten minutes a day.

To re-cap, the following are crucial:

- Having a clear goal

- Relaxing your mind

- Visualising with emotion as if you have already achieved your goal

- Connecting with others (either electronically, personally or in book form)

- Making a daily action-plan so that you can achieve your goal (mini-steps are easily achievable)

- Making adjustments to achieve your goals (remembering to exercise on most days and relax at least once daily)

- Do not self-sabotage by using old, unhelpful habits or patterns (such as being negative) rather, create new . helpful ones

- Use this technique (of utilising helpful patterns) for your life-long visions as well as daily ones (for example: affirming, 'I have plenty of finances, robust all-round wellness, inter-connected supportive and caring relationships)

- Do not get over-tired, have adequate sleep and keep your goals in mind

The main issue about managing time is planning your daily schedule around priorities. These include your personal life. Each priority needs to be stated by you so that activities can relate to personal as well as work issues. By doing this, more time can be spent on what needs to be achieved and less time on what is not a priority.

When time managing, be specific regarding your needs for buffering against anxiety, as already explained.

Just as a reminder: on a daily basis, sleep adequately, eat healthily, hydrate by drinking water, physically move for at least twenty minutes, rest by relaxing, and dream the goal you wish for, relax and connect with at least one other person such as a relative. Do whatever you spend a substantial amount of time doing on most days while awake, such as housekeeping or composing, with a positive attitude. Allocate time realistically for all these situations and you can experience anxiety melting away.

Remember to help yourself in what seem like obvious ways; but so many people do not do them: Have proper meals daily, take a walk in the fresh air and do enough exercise. Face that phobia in the way I explained earlier and it disappears! Steer away from unhelpful behaviour.

Chapter 18 Setting Goals

Anxiety management tactics we covered so far are great in a short and middle term. Continuous dedication and adoption of these tactics into your daily routine will eliminate panic attacks and reduce your anxiety but getting your anxiety under control permanently requires further work. Long term anxiety management requires analysis, review and alteration of how you perceive the world around you.

Anxiety management is an ongoing process that requires diligence and determination. To keep your eyes on the prize you will set goals you want to achieve. Setting goals is a great exercise as it diverts your efforts and gives your endeavors purpose.

Without a specific, articulated purpose you can spend a lot of time and waste a lot of effort without any significant result. Water can fall on the ground harmlessly or it can break any barrier. If you are not focused on your effort, your effort will bear no fruit like water falling harmlessly during the rain. It takes concentrated effort and determination to achieve your goals.

Your actions require a clear purpose which is specific enough. It is not enough to tell yourself that you want to be happy. What happiness means to you?

We all have limited resources and one resource which we have to take into account the most is time. Time is the reason why you can not afford to have vague goals in your life because you will only end up always lagging behind, trying to catch up to a number of goals which are slipping away.

This is a great source of anxiety on its own. Setting clear priorities will eliminate conflicts that you have to deal with on a daily basis. You will have guidelines for your life you can use to make quick and clear decisions.

My priorities in life, in order of their significance, are family, health and my career. Having clear priorities removes anxiety that stems from indecision or second-guessing.

Setting goals has another great effect - having clear goals gives you additional strength. People were able to overcome insurmountable obstacles to achieve their goals. Goals you feel passionate about will give you powerful motivation and a feeling that you can achieve anything.

Keep these goals always in your sight. You can put them on your fridge or on your bathroom mirror so it is the first thing you see every day. Share your goals with people closest to you. They will provide you with support and help you achieve your goals.

Take a moment to think about what are your main priorities in life. Write them down in an order of their importance. Do not set more than five priorities as not to dilute your attention.

MY MAIN PRIORITIES

1.

2.

3.

4.

5.

Now that you have your priorities straight you can make plans and set goals. Write down a short story about your typical day after you end this program without fear and worry controlling your life. Give this story tangibility by adding details. Create a short movie with your words about your day starting with you waking up and ending with you falling asleep happy and without any difficulty.

Focus on events as they happen and your feelings now that you are not under the thumb of anxiety. Be sure to include your new healthy habits.

Review your story and note events and feelings. For example, you might have written that you had to do a presentation in front of an important client and you felt calm, confident and persuasive. Details in your story uncover your desires. Use these to help you write up to five goals you set yourself for the next two weeks.

TWO WEEK GOALS

1.

2.

3.

4.

5.

    Write down goals you set for yourself for half a year. Two week goals have to be as specific as you can make them. Your goals for the middle term can be less specific but avoid being too vague.

SIX MONTH GOALS

1.

2.

3.

4.

5.

    Finally you need to set yourself long term goals. These goals reflect your main values and priorities.

LONG TERM GOALS

1.

2.

3.

Goals, even long term, are not meant to remain constant. Review and update your goals constantly to keep them relevant. This is especially true for short term goals.

Use these goals to give you drive to grow and improve yourself and to achieve happiness you deserve. Earl Nightingale stressed the importance of having clear goals, "People with goals succeed because they know where they are going."

Chapter 19 Herbal and Vitamin Remedies

Before you consider adding any of the following herbs or vitamins, consult with your doctor. They can warn you about any potential interactions they can have with medications you are on and talk to you about whether or not they are right for you.

Kampo

This is a traditional Japanese medication that is used to treat a variety of things. It is based on conventional Chinese medication. The underlying concept of this set of therapeutic medicine and different theories is that there has to be harmony between physical and mental health. There is no separation between the two. Kampo treatment generally includes things like acupuncture, but some herbs are taken to reduce anxiety. Kami-shoyo-shan and Hange-kobuko-to are both medicines that have been shown to overcome panic attacks and anxiety. Again, ask your doctor before adding this to your routine.

Kava Kava

This is a Polynesian plant that is well-known for its calming effects. Kava kava has been used by the natives of the South Pacific Islands for centuries as a type of medicine. It is particularly useful for those who experience mild to moderate levels of anxiety. In addition to anxiety, it can be useful in treating sleeplessness and restlessness. There are several things to consider before taking kava. It cannot be combined with alcohol or psychotropic medications.

Inositol

This is a carbohydrate supplement. It comes in a powder form. It has been proven to help people with panic attacks. Inositol is a naturally occurring substance in your body that helps in cell formation. It is also thought to affect the action of the neurotransmitter serotonin. Your level of serotonin can affect feelings of anxiety and depression.

Chamomile

Chamomile is a daisy-like plant that originally grew in Europe. Chamomile tea has long been thought to have soothing effects on people. Some of the compounds in chamomile bind to the same brain receptors as drugs like Valium. If you know you are going into a stressful situation, a cup of chamomile tea may help you feel calmer. It can also be taken in supplement form.

Valerian

The most important thing to note about valerian is it WILL make you sleepy. It can be used to help you get the recommended 8 hours of sleep at night. If you experience a lot of anxiety around bedtime, this may be an herbal supplement for you. It is not something you would want to take before heading to work. Valerian acts as a sedative in both the brain and the nervous system. Side effects are rare but can include headaches and a feeling of sluggishness the next morning. In rare cases, it may have the opposite effect on a person and cause excitability and insomnia.

Lemon Balm

Sold as a tea, capsule, and tincture (a medicine made by dissolving a drug in alcohol,) lemon balm has been used since at least the Middle Ages to reduce stress and anxiety. It also helps with sleep. Lemon balm contains chemicals that seem to act as a sedative, creating a calming effect. Potential side effects include dizziness, nausea, and vomiting. Be aware that some studies suggest that taking too much can actually cause more anxiety, so it would be wise to start with the smallest possible dose and see how you react.

Lavender

This is something you would want to use aromatically, not orally. The scent of lavender is thought to be intoxicating while being calming. It is often used in doctor and dentist waiting rooms to help keep patients calm while they wait to be seen. Buying a few lavender-scented candles or bubble bath and using them at home may help foster an overall feeling of calmness.

Ashwagandha

This is a popular herb with many benefits. It is known to protect the nervous system as well as reduce anxiety. If that wasn't enough, it also is a potent immune-system booster. It should be used in combination with deep breathing and an improved diet. Taking a hefty dose of ashwagandha can cause vomiting, diarrhea, and a generally upset stomach. As with any herbal supplement, discuss it with your doctor before adding it to your routine. It should NOT be taken when pregnant and could negatively impact those with diabetes.

Brahmi

Also known as Gotu Kola, it has long been used to treat a variety of things in Indian medicine. It decreases blood pressure in veins. Not only has it been used to treat anxiety, but it is also used to improve cognitive function as well. It is believed to improve the impulse transmission between nerve cells in the brain. Studies have even shown it to raise IQ and improve concentration. As a bonus, it increases the all-important serotonin levels in the brain, fostering a feeling of relaxation and a reduction in anxiety.

Ginkgo Biloba

The uses of Ginkgo Biloba are incredibly varied. It has been shown that an extract of ginkgo Biloba took for 4 weeks can be useful in reducing anxiety. Many of the health benefits of ginkgo Biloba are aimed at the mind, and it is a popular treatment for Alzheimer's disease and other forms of dementia. It is possible to be allergic to Ginkgo Biloba, and people who are allergic to poison ivy, poison oak, or cashew shell oil should be particularly careful.

Conclusion

Trying to adjust to a reality that isn't ideal can be difficult for some people, but it is something that needs to be done to be able to overcome anxiety and depression. People who are able to overcome it are those who want to make sure that they are doing the right thing and that they are not the victim of their past. By looking at the past and overcoming it, reality therapy is able to change the way that the present is handled. People who choose to overcome it will no longer be victims of their past but will, instead, be able to flourish in their new role as someone who has defeated an anxiety or depression disorder.

Right and Wrong

The first thing that reality therapy will focus on is whether or not something is right or wrong. The therapy aims to take a look at the way that things can change and the different aspects of it. The person should decide whether something is right or wrong.

When using reality therapy, the person needs to listen to their own inner voice. Most are surprised to find that it is difficult to think of what they believe instead of what they have been told to believe or what they have been told is right or wrong. This is something that will change the way that they do things, though, and it will give them a better chance at doing more for themselves. When they are able to use their own inner voice instead of the voice of someone else who has told them how to think, they will be able to make a decision on what is right and what is wrong.

The easiest way to do this is to create a list of things that are in the moral gray area. The list can be anything that is close to them or related to them, but it should be something that has strong moral implications. When the person looks at it, they should decide the black and white area that the previously gray area item went into. It is something that will change depending on the situation, and it will give them a new perspective on the way that they should feel about things instead of just going off of whatever they have been told to feel.

Responsibility

When a person experiences anxiety or depression, they may feel like they can place the blame on something or someone else. The biggest thing that they need to be able to do is learn how to take responsibility for their own mental illness. It can be difficult, but it is something that can be done with a little bit of practice.

To be able to take responsibility of their mental disorder, they need to look at the whys of having it. Do they think that they have it from their parents? Because they had a traumatic youth? Because they don't know how to function in social situations? By looking at each of these reasons, it is clear to see that they are putting the blame on something other than themselves.

It can be really difficult to get to this point, but it is a good thing once it happens. If a person is able to look at themselves and say: "I have depression as a result of my own brain reacting differently" they will then be able to take care of the problem and make sure that they are fixing their depression.

The difference in responsibility and blame is that a person who is responsible for something aims to fix the problem that is currently happening. A person who is blaming someone for their problems will not want to fix the current problem but will, instead, be focused on the problems of their past. They will want to blame these people for the problems that they have.

Realism

Understanding the way that the world works is one of the most important qualities that come along with trying to make reality therapy work. The person who has anxiety or depression may be stuck in the past in their own head, and that is something that can be a problem. By taking a step back and looking at the different things that can be done in the present, they are going to give themselves a better chance at reality. It is a great way for people to make sure that they are getting the most out of reality and that they are able to provide themselves with the best opportunity possible.

The easiest way to do this is to keep track of each of the things that are actually going on. A person should write down the different positive things that are happening in their daily lives.

By keeping track of this, they can, essentially, pull themselves out from the muck that is in the past and can be holding them down. It is a good idea to make sure that the things they are focusing on, in reality, are positive.

By making sure that they know what is going on with reality and that things are happening all around them, they will have a better chance at moving on from the past, doing the right thing and joining everyone in reality.

Overcoming It

Each of these methods can make reality therapy truly work for anyone who is suffering from anxiety or depression. It is one of the easiest therapy options regarding logistics, but it can be hard for people to make sure that they are truly pulling themselves out of the past. Because of the problems that come with the different therapy methods, people may want to choose reality as a way to make sure that they are doing things the right way.

While it may be uncomfortable to focus on the present instead of the past, it is one of the first steps of healing. With reality therapy, people can make sure that they are getting the most out of each situation and that they are doing the best job possible at becoming a better, happier person.

Reality therapy does not always work the way that you want it to. It may take some extra time and may be a problem for people who are in different situations. It can be extremely detrimental for people to think that they are going to be able to do different things in a world that is truly real, instead of thinking about the different ways that they will not be able to do things. Because of this, a person should always be cautious when they are using reality therapy. It can be painful to look at the past and overcome it, but it can also be beneficial for people who want to be able to do more with the past and with the different things that they have going on at the present time.

www.ingramcontent.com/pod-product-compliance
Lightning Source LLC
Chambersburg PA
CBHW021420210526
45463CB00001B/470